"A well needed exploration of unconscious work and theories about it, at once thoughtful, creative, evocative. Aspects of the Jungian, Relational, and Lacanian unconscious are viewed from an interpersonal perspective. The authors leave the way open for diverse approaches to interact and enrich each other, pulsating with possibilities. Rather than tying everything up, the book feels like a beginning through which we speak with the unconscious speaking with us."

Michael Eigen, *The Challenge of Being Human*,
The Sensitive Self, *Feeling Matters*, and *Flames from the*
Unconscious: Trauma, Madness, Faith

"Though unconscious process and unconscious motivation has been at the center of psychoanalytic thinking from its inception, there has been only minimal literature comparing different ways of thinking about these key concepts that have evolved beyond Freud's original description and its ego-psychological emendations. This scholarly and well written volume brings us up-to-date, delineating key contemporary conceptualizations of unconscious process, comparing them with each other as well as with Freudian theorizing. It should be required reading for anyone interested in psychoanalysis."

Irwin Hirsch, Ph.D., NYU Postdoctoral Program
in Psychotherapy and Psychoanalysis; the Wm. Alanson White
Institute; the Manhattan Institute for Psychoanalysis

"A book full of enriching analyses of the so called 'vast domain'—the unconscious. A must for everyone entangled in the discourse on psychoanalysis and those who want to get involved."

Rosemarie Brucher is a scholar in Theater Studies
and Vice-Rector of Research at the Music and
Arts University of the City of Vienna

"A rich and rewarding collection of essays that expands our understanding and appreciation of the unconscious. Drawing on a diversity of voices and opinions, the editors weave a tapestry of viewpoints that challenge standard assumptions about the nature of unconscious experience and its applications. With themes ranging from the intrapsychic and the implicit, to language and symbolism, sexuality and gender, race and social class, this important new volume provides essential insights on the unconscious."

Roger Frie, Professor of Education, Simon Fraser
University and Affiliate Professor of Psychiatry,
University of British Columbia

T0386183

The Unconscious

This book explores the unconscious in psychoanalysis using cross-disciplinary input from cultural, social, and linguistic perspectives. This book is the first contemporary collection applying the various perspectives from within the psychoanalytic discipline.

It covers the unconscious from three main perspectives: the metaphysical, including links with quantum mechanics and Jung's thought; the socio-relational, drawing on ideas from politics, inter-generational trauma, and the interpersonal; and the linguistic, drawing on notions of the social construct of language and hermeneutics. Throughout the history of psychoanalysis, theorists have wrestled with the ubiquitousness and diverse nature of the unconscious. This collection is an account of the contemporary psychoanalytic struggle to understand and work with this quintessential, defining, and foundational object of psychoanalysis.

This book is primarily of interest to practicing clinicians and trainees. It is also of significant interest to any academic professionals and students who adapt psychoanalytic thought in their studies in the humanities, including literature, philosophy, and the social sciences.

Pascal Sauvayre is a member of the faculty and a training and supervising analyst at the William Alanson White Institute. He has a private practice in New York City. He is a co-translator of the upcoming translation of Laplanche's *The Tub: Transcendence of the Transference*.

David Braucher is a member of the faculty of the William Alanson White Institute's Division I Psychoanalytic Program and a lecturer at NYU Steinhart. He is on the editorial board of the journal, *Contemporary Psychoanalysis*, and author of Life Smarts on PsychologyToday.com. He is in private practice in Manhattan's West Village.

Psychoanalysis in a new key book series
Donnel Stern
Series Editor

When music is played in a new key, the melody does not change, but the notes that make up the composition do: change in the context of continuity, continuity that perseveres through change. Psychoanalysis in a New Key publishes books that share the aims psychoanalysts have always had, but that approach them differently. The books in the series are not expected to advance any particular theoretical agenda, although to this date most have been written by analysts from the Interpersonal and Relational orientations.

The most important contribution of a psychoanalytic book is the communication of something that nudges the reader's grasp of clinical theory and practice in an unexpected direction. Psychoanalysis in a New Key creates a deliberate focus on innovative and unsettling clinical thinking. Because that kind of thinking is encouraged by exploration of the sometimes surprising contributions to psychoanalysis of ideas and findings from other fields, Psychoanalysis in a New Key particularly encourages interdisciplinary studies. Books in the series have married psychoanalysis with dissociation, trauma theory, sociology, and criminology. The series is open to the consideration of studies examining the relationship between psychoanalysis and any other field—for instance, biology, literary and art criticism, philosophy, systems theory, anthropology, and political theory.

But innovation also takes place within the boundaries of psychoanalysis, and Psychoanalysis in a New Key therefore also presents work that reformulates thought and practice without leaving the precincts of the field. Books in the series focus, for example, on the significance of personal values in psychoanalytic practice, on the complex interrelationship between the analyst's clinical work and personal life, on the consequences for the clinical situation when patient and analyst are from different cultures, and on the need for psychoanalysts to accept the degree to which they knowingly satisfy their own wishes during treatment hours, often to the patient's detriment. A full list of all titles in this series is available at: https://www.routledge.com/series/LEAPNKBS

The Unconscious

Contemporary Refractions In Psychoanalysis

Edited by Pascal Sauvayre and
David Braucher

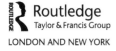
Routledge
Taylor & Francis Group

LONDON AND NEW YORK

First published 2021
by Routledge
2 Park Square, Milton Park, Abingdon, Oxon OX14 4RN

and by Routledge
52 Vanderbilt Avenue, New York, NY 10017

Routledge is an imprint of the Taylor & Francis Group, an informa business

British Library Cataloguing-in-Publication Data
A catalogue record for this book is available from the British Library

Library of Congress Cataloging-in-Publication Data
A catalog record has been requested for this book

ISBN: 978-0-367-49841-2 (hbk)
ISBN: 978-0-367-49839-9 (pbk)
ISBN: 978-1-003-04764-3 (ebk)

Typeset in Times
by Deanta Global Publishing Services, Chennai, India

Contents

Contributors

David Braucher has been a practicing clinician for over 25 years. He is a member of the faculty of the William Alanson White Institute's Division I Psychoanalytic Program and a lecturer at NYU Steinhart. He is on the editorial board of the journal *Contemporary Psychoanalysis*, and he is the executive editor of the blog Contemporary Psychoanalysis in Action. He is the author of Life Smarts on PsychologyToday.com. He is in private practice in the West Village/Chelsea neighborhood of Manhattan.

Burton Budick received an AB degree from Harvard College in 1959. He earned a doctoral degree from UC Berkeley in 1962. He was a postdoc and then an instructor at Columbia University Physics Department from 1962 to 1964. He spent 1964 to 1968 at the Hebrew University in Jerusalem, Israel. From 1968 until the present he has been an associate and full professor at New York University, specializing in nuclear and particle physics.

Jonathan House splits his time between clinical work, teaching at Columbia's Institute for Comparative Literature and Society—Freud in the Fall; Laplanche in the Spring—and working for The Unconscious in Translation, where he has translated, co-translated, and/or edited translations of the work of Jean Laplanche, Dominique Scarfone, J.-B. Pontalis, Hélène Tessier, and others. He was appointed by Laplanche to the Conseil Scientifique of Fondation Laplanche, where he is responsible for the English translations.

Orsi Hunyady is a clinical psychologist and psychoanalyst working in private practice in New York City. She is on faculty at the Clinical

Internship Program at Adelphi University and the Adult Psychoanalytic Training Program at the William Alanson White Institute (WAWI). She is supervising at Adelphi University and in the Intensive Psychoanalytic Psychotherapy Program (IPPP) of WAWI. She is an associate editor for the journal of *Contemporary Psychoanalysis*, and author of several articles in the field of psychoanalysis.

Ruth Imber is a training and supervising analyst and Fellow Emeritus at the William Alanson White Institute where she is Director of the Appointments and Promotions Committee. She is a member of the editorial board of the journal *Contemporary Psychoanalysis*. She has published papers and book chapters on pregnancy, parenting, and aspects of psychoanalytic theory. She treats adults and couples in New York City.

Lynne Layton is a psychoanalyst and on the faculty of Harvard Medical School. She supervises at the Massachusetts Institute for Psychoanalysis and is adjunct faculty at Pacifica Graduate Institute. She is the author of *Who's That Girl? Who's That Boy? Clinical Practice Meets Postmodern Gender Theory*, co-editor of *Bringing the Plague. Toward a Postmodern Psychoanalysis*, and co-editor of *Psychoanalysis, Class and Politics: Encounters in the Clinical Setting*. She is editor emeritus of the journal *Psychoanalysis, Culture & Society*, associate editor of *Studies in Gender and Sexuality*, and co-founder of the Boston Psychosocial Work Group. She is Past-President of Section IX, Psychoanalysis for Social Responsibility, of Division 39, and co-founder of Reflective Spaces/Material Places, Boston.

Michael Monhart is a candidate at the Jungian Psychoanalytical Association in New York City. He is the author of "The Path of Individuation in Shingon Buddhism" in the forthcoming Proceedings of the 2016 Congress of the International Association for Analytical Psychology. He also works as a Tibetan translator and is the co-editor and translator of the short stories of the Tibetan author Pema Tseden to be published as *Enticements* (SUNY 2018).

Katharina Rothe is a clinical psychologist, psychoanalyst, and psychosocial researcher. She is a graduate of psychoanalytic training and a member of faculty at the W. A. White Institute and maintains a private practice in New York City. She is widely published in academic journals and books on psychoanalysis, qualitative methods in psychoanalytic social research, sex and gender, anti-Semitism, racism, and the aftermath of National Socialism (Monograph: Rothe, K. (2009). *Das (Nicht-) Sprechen über die Judenvernichtung. Psychische Weiterwirkungen des Holocaust in mehreren Generationen nicht-jüdischer Deutscher. Gießen: Psychosozial.*) She is a co-editor of the German journal *Psychoanalyse. Texte zur Sozialforschung* [Psychoanalysis. Contributions to Social Research] and an associate editor of *Contemporary Psychoanalysis*.

Avgi Saketopoulou is a psychoanalyst based in New York City and a graduate of the New York University Postdoctoral Program in Psychotherapy and Psychoanalysis. She is on the editorial boards of the *Journal of the American Psychoanalytic Association, Studies in Gender and Sexuality*, and *Psychoanalytic Dialogues* and has spoken and published widely on sexuality, gender, class, and race. Dr. Saketopoulou received several prizes for her writing, including the Ruth Stein Prize and in 2014 the Ralph Roughton Award from the American Psychoanalytic Association. She is on the faculty of the Stephen Mitchell Relational Study Center, the National Institute for the Psychotherapies (NIP), the New York University Postdoctoral Program in Psychotherapy and Psychoanalysis, the New York Psychoanalytic Institute, and the W. A. White Institute.

Pascal Sauvayre is a training and supervising analyst and a member of faculty at the William Alanson White Institute. He is an executive editor for *Contemporary Psychoanalysis* and he studies and writes at the disciplinary boundaries of psychoanalysis. He has a practice in New York City.

Daniel Shaw is a psychoanalyst in private practice in New York City and in Nyack, New York; and a faculty member and supervisor at the National Institute for the Psychotherapies in New York. His papers have appeared in *Psychoanalytic Inquiry, Contemporary Psychoanalysis*, and *Psychoanalytic Dialogues*, and most recently, his book *Traumatic Narcissism: Relational Systems of Subjugation* was published by Routledge for the Relational Perspectives Series.

Donnel B. Stern is a Training and Supervising Analyst at the William Alanson White Institute in New York City; Clinical Professor and Clinical Consultant at the New York University Postdoctoral Program in Psychoanalysis and Psychotherapy; and a member of the faculty at the New York Psychoanalytic Institute. He is the editor of Psychoanalysis in a New Key, a book series at Routledge, and is the former Editor-in-Chief of *Contemporary Psychoanalysis*. He has co-edited four books and authored four others, the most recent of which is *The Infinity of the Unsaid: Unformulated Experience, Language, and the Nonverbal* (2018). He serves as an associate editor or on the editorial boards of a number of psychoanalytic journals. Dr. Stern is in private practice in New York City.

Warren Wilner is a faculty member, training analyst, and supervising analyst at the William Alanson White Institute; faculty member and supervising consultant at the New York University Postdoctoral Program; author of some 25 published papers in psychoanalysis, with an emphasis on the experiential nature of the analytic process; and has a private practice in New York City.

Introduction

Pascal Sauvayre and David Braucher

The idea for this collection emerged over the course of a yearlong colloquium series on the topic of 'the Unconscious,' sponsored by the White Society over the 2017–2018 academic year. This issue is a collection of those papers accompanied by the discussants' commentaries.

Early on in the series, we marveled over the inventiveness and creativity involved in theorizing this quintessential analytic object. The differences that immediately came to the fore were not just a matter of different approaches, but differences in terminologies, in vocabularies. And yet, the liveliness of the discussions also pointed to the possibility of an enriching discourse. A clear thread linking the different approaches emerged, and following it led naturally to this collection.

Can these theories interact and enrich each other? We believe that this book takes on this challenge and answers affirmatively. In his paper, Monhart clearly expresses the rationale for this collection even before it was conceived, "this colloquium series is so important—it at once takes us back to our roots of working with the unconscious and allows us all to compare maps, and through dialogue, gain shared knowledge of this inner world." Indeed, we believe that we are called upon to develop a modicum of fluency in multiple 'idiolects.' Stern explains that "to describe theories as idiolects is to emphasize diversity (each theory's unique purview) within an underlying unity (the broader 'language' that defines psychoanalysis)."

Freud initially took an overlooked idea that had been lying around the intellectual landscape and gave it a name: the unconscious. Although, at the time, it was beginning to gain some attention, it was Freud who put it at the very epicenter of the human drama. Freud's own thinking about the unconscious was slippery and polyvalent: he sometimes referred to it as a site, an organ, a process, a function, a force, a thing, and a location, among others.

From Freud's initial forays, the concept quickly refracted, like white light shot through a prism; each new theory, like a photon, following the trajectory of its unique wavelength, taking its place in the spectrum's continuum. In particular, the presence of the 'other,' conceived in different ways, from the metaphysical, to the socio-political, and the linguistic, seems to provide the contemporary prism through which the unconscious is being refracted. Depending on the psychoanalytic theory to which it is being applied, the concept of the unconscious becomes formulated through the languages and idiolects of those theories.

As the presentations proceeded, and with the privilege of retrospection, it began to dawn on us, dare we say 'après-coup,' that there was really something unique here—each new paper, in discourse with the others, like the spectrum's colors blending at the edges, expanded the possibilities of thought. The relevance of this collection of papers became clear as each perspective was enriched when considered with the other papers and commentaries in the series.

But this book also takes on the complementary task of tracing the common thread present in all psychoanalytic approaches, which is to ground the different theories in human experience and practice. Indeed, all of the papers' theoretical considerations are grounded in human experience, whether it be in literature, in personal experience, or in clinical material. Throughout the history of psychoanalysis, this dilemma—the unconscious' ubiquitousness and diversity—has been a central challenge: how does one reconcile the richly divergent conceptualizations with their common roots in human experience and praxis? This collection is an account of some contemporary struggles to understand and work with this quintessential, defining, and foundational source-object of psychoanalysis: the unconscious.

The first part looks at the unconscious from the vantage point of its convergence with the 'other-world' of the metaphysical. Wilner launches the reader beyond the foundations of time and space of our world into an exploration of the unconscious as an event that occurs out of time, now-here, and is always out of place, nowhere. Using the 'quantum dilemma' as a launching pad, his 'no-where'/'now-here' house of mirrors illustrates the simultaneous elusiveness and ubiquitousness of how lived unconscious experience 'takes us' 'outside' of time into the immediacy of the now-here "of merged relational events that are going on 'presently,' which is to say timelessly 'within it.'" In his discussion, Budick delves deeper into the mystery of relativity, adding Einstein's 'elsewhere' to Wilner's 'no-where' and 'now-here,' further demonstrating the intersection between psychoanalytic thought and quantum theory.

Notwithstanding these complex theoretical considerations, Wilner never allows us to get lost in speculative physics. Using compelling material from his clinical practice, including the fascinating metaphor of the unconscious as the Lone Ranger, Wilner evokes rather than explains the elusive, polysemic, and polymorphous nature of the unconscious. As Wilner posits, "the very act of directly trying to make the unconscious conscious, a hallowed goal of psychoanalytic practice, may be, like a cat trying to chase its own tail, to actually create more unconscious flux."

Monhart then grapples with Jung's more mystical elsewhere. Emphasizing how working with the unconscious is an avenue allowing for passage between the personal to the collective, Monhart takes many of Jung's fundamental concepts (including the structure of the psyche, the complexes, the personal and collective unconscious, archetypes, symbol formation and interpretation in symptoms and dreams, psychic energy, synchronicity, and the prospective aspect of individuation) and tracks the 'other's' presence in the intersubjective tightrope between the personal and collective. Monhart's discussion of dreams (his patients' and Jung's) is then deepened in Shaw's commentary illustrating the potential power of the unconscious to "achieve a modicum of communion with the world at large."

It is interesting here to pause and reflect on the other-worldly presence of Jung's collective unconscious and track the links to the characteristics of the unconscious that exceed the space-time continuum—both showing how the unconscious stretches beyond our conventional human dimensions.

The second part delves into the relational nature of the unconscious as it manifests in shared experiences from the dyadic intimacy of the analytic setting to the internalized influences of the socio-political environment in which we live. It highlights unconscious processes as they manifest in enactments that pervade all of our relationships from those we have with personal others in our lives to the relationship we have with socio-political structures and mytho-symbolic narratives.

Providing a critique of Benjamin's 'analytic third' and 'doer and done to' concepts, Imber examines the intersubjective approach to the unconscious from an interpersonal perspective. Considering the ubiquity of unconscious enactments that persist in interpersonal relating, we are forever becoming aware of them after the fact—if ever; there is always an aspect of our relating which remains unconscious. In critiquing Benjamin's intersubjective approach, Imber cautions clinicians to be aware of the limitations of their conscious understanding and the importance of honoring patients' need for separateness. She encourages clinicians to avoid quickly smoothing over interpersonal anger and to remain attentive to the need to maintain private inner worlds.

Braucher expands on this discussion of enactments in the clinical situation by exploring how it is influenced by the mytho-symbolic narratives of the patriarchy and fatherhood and how this aspect of the unconscious is pertinent to understanding the current socio-political situation. Building off of Freud's 'paternal principle,' Kohut's 'idealizing selfobject' and Lacan's 'Le Nom du Père,' Braucher explores how the father is largely a transference phenomenon enacted by the child. Providing examples from life, literature, and the cinema, he expands the notion of the 'paternal principle' arguing for the 'power principle,' that is, how the child imbues the father with his power, rendering him paradoxically in a vulnerable position.

Considering that the father's power is dependent on the child's perception of him as powerful, the child is free to eventually attribute that same power to others, rendering the original father obsolete. Using clinical examples, he shows how, despite a patriarchy in decline, the patriarch of the father's own childhood remains as an unconscious 'paternal bastion' holding men accountable to this archaic and patriarchic ideal, while no longer being perceived as powerful by his children and without the support of the patriarchal systems of the past.

Layton elaborates on unconscious psychosocial processes that permeate identity formation and clinical work and how "intergenerational transmission of trauma creates a normative unconscious." She demonstrates how racist, sexist, and classist enactments in the clinic are examples of normative unconscious processes that maintain cultural and power inequalities. The identities of patients and therapists are formed by cultural demands to split off and project aspects of their humanity that fail to conform to positions in society. "[R]acism and class inequality do not only split the psyche of the subordinate; they also bolster the fantasmatic position of the dominant—and BOTH parties want to hold to the fantasy that SOMEONE is invulnerable to pain and loss." The chapter concludes with thoughts about contemporary social forces that contribute to White middle-class subject formation and White middle-class symptoms, focusing again on unconscious collusions that stem from both culture and clinic.

In her commentary, Rothe contrasts Layton's concept of the *normative unconscious* with essential aspects of Freud's unconscious highlighting the importance of an unconscious apart from unconscious processes. While she cautions against the "risk of reifying it ... the German Marxist term for reification (being): Verdinglichung, literally: 'thinging-it'," she observes that

> [n]o matter how hard we try to analyze the social processes we are ourselves entangled in, we also imbue them with something more, this layer of fantasy—including unconscious fantasy—the kind of surplus that thinkers of 'the unconscious' have been trying to capture.

This 'surplus' is precisely a concept that will be developed in the third part.

It is fascinating to consider the chapters of the second part together. They take the reader through a back and forth process between the personal and the social dimensions of the unconscious, both within and between each of the chapters. Keeping the tension between the personal and the social is essential to good psychoanalytic practice and theorizing. But one can also see the threads linking to the other-worldliness of the collective unconscious, of the supra-personal and the metaphysical. Indeed, this comparison helps us in the most difficult passage between the different levels of the personal, social, and supra-personal, not by establishing a clear cut or dogmatic system, but by floating between different vocabularies and by allowing, or indeed challenging, the reader to open his/her mind to alternative discourses. This challenge brings us precisely to the topic of the third part, the unconscious through the prism of language.

The third part concerns some of the most influential contemporary theorizers of the unconscious, and it takes on the challenge of shifting discourses on different levels. It begins with Sauvayre and Hunyady's take on one of the central themes of this book by attempting a comparative study in psychoanalysis of two apparently dissimilar theories. Although Sullivan and Lacan have vastly different approaches to Freud's language, their similarities, as well as their possibilities for enriching each other, emerge. Using a close reading of each theorist's lived experience, the authors show how one can move from one idiolect to the other.

Stern explicates how describing the theories as idiolects emphasizes their differences while acknowledging their shared foundation in a common psychoanalytic language. But he cautions that with each transition from one language to another "there is a loss of information, so to speak, as there used to be, in the old days before digital recording, when you transferred sound from vinyl records to audiotape, or images from film to videotape."

Next, House explores Laplanche's central concept of translation of the 'implanted enigmatic message,' the 'surplus' of which takes us by surprise and defines the analytic object, the unconscious. It is this 'surplus,' untranslated or untranslatable, that inspires the individual to attempt, 'après-coup' to formulate its meaning. We can find some fascinating links between Layton's exploration of "the normative unconscious processes as effects of an intergenerational transmission of trauma" and House's exploration of Laplanche's 'implantation of the enigmatic message.'

Saketopoulo, deepening the combined meaning of 'après-coup' as both deferred action and retrospective modification, posits that

> it is only the portion of the unconscious that can hook itself onto the mytho-symbolic narratives widely circulating in culture, that can develop escape velocity to make it out of the inchoate so that it may be churned into some rudimentary form of meaning.

She further explores these narratives in the sociopolitics of the #MeToo movement, raising interesting questions about the links between the notion of the 'normative unconscious' explored in Part II and the dialogical scripts analyzed here.

The challenges of translation, with the risks of impoverishment and the rewards of enrichment, are found in all aspects of this book. House quotes Eco on the translations of his own work.

> Note that the English version is snappier than the Italian, and perhaps someday, on making a revised edition of my novel, I might use the English formula rather than the Italian. Would we then say that I have

changed my text? We certainly would. Thus, the English translation is a failed translation of the Italian. In spite of this, the English text says exactly what I wanted to say.

Our hope is that moving about these different idiolects does not simply lead us to speak broken or impoverished Jungian, or Laplanchian, and so forth. Rather, in Eco's spirit, it helps the reader focus on a specific term, or issue, or a specific formulation of the unconscious, and use complementary, or even competing ones to enrich their own. Another hope is that the theorizing in the following pages generates further thought.

While we celebrate the theoretical diversity in the following pages, it is absolutely essential to note that what makes all psychoanalytic theorizing unique is its reliance on clinical experience. All of the following papers rely on such experience, whether it be of a biographical, autobiographical, or fictional nature. Sullivan haunted by a spider, Lacan being awakened by the knocks, Jung's discussions with Philemon, Wilner's missing hands, Braucher's weeping father, differing translations of *The Odyssey*, and Layton's use of her niece Emily's short film trilogy *Lovestruck* are just a few of the fascinating representations of human experience upon which these theoretical formulations are rooted.

In Part I, Monhart emphasizes how this series of papers connects us to our common roots in working with the unconscious and allows us to share different perceptions, expanding our understanding of this source-object of psychoanalysis. We conclude with Saketopoulo, pointing us toward the future and the continued theorizing of these central psychoanalytic concepts, "we should all be looking forward to tracking how they will be taken up by other analytic scholars and to the innovative analytic theorizing they can ignite in our field," perhaps in a new book of this nature.

Part I

The unconscious is everywhere, and nowhere

Chapter I

From out of nowhere—The paradox of unconscious experience[1]

Warren Wilner

Unique analyst that he was—and promulgating the concept of psychic uniqueness as he did—Ben Wolstein (1982) had many creative takes on theoretical and clinical psychoanalysis. But one idea that has passed relatively unnoticed (and, to my regret, I never asked him more about it while he was alive) was his frequent reference to the apparent paradox of unconscious experience. If something is unconscious, how can it be experienced? Wolstein considered such experience, should we find it to actually exist, to be private and not shareable.

I think of the unconscious much like the past is described in Jack Finney's delightful novel *Time and Again* (1970/1995): it's always with us, its expressions always potentially present in awareness. We are kept in the conscious present, in part—according to Finney—by the environmental cues that reinforce for us being in this reality. As Wittgenstein has said, a picture holds us captive, and keeps repeating itself to us over and over again (as cited in Finch, 1977). Finney fancifully suggests that if these cues were to dramatically change, we could conceivably be catapulted by a kind of quantum leap back into a specific past or—as I in a loosely analogous way consider here—into an eternal unconscious present. Implicit in Finney's idea is that there is a link between the psychic and physical worlds. Here, I use the concept of unconscious experience in order to explore this idea.

My intention is to go beyond a characterization and description of a concept of unconscious experience, and to provide—through clinical and other life examples, as well as by psychoanalytic, philosophical, linguistic, and literary reference—fresh perspectives on what the nature and structure of unconscious experience might be. I also seek to explore a possible connection between the psychic and physical worlds to which Finney alludes in his novel. Fundamental to this study will be the distinction between experience and what is happening in the physical world, in reality. In order to establish a strong basis in the physical world for this comparison, I lean heavily on some fascinating findings and theories in physics that offer, by way of metaphor and possible direct correspondence, a model or graphic picture of what the dimension of unconscious experience may be, and what we might consider to be 'the unconscious' itself.

The unconscious is nowhere

Since time immemorial, we have tried to account for psychical phenomena that seem to come from out of nowhere. Wolstein (Personal Communication, 1975) said that he considered such phenomena to be emanations from the unconscious. He describes these as intrusions of the unconscious. In a different vein, Kabbalists talk about the Kabalistic god, the Ein Sof, which is not god the creator. Rather, the Kabalistic vision is of a hidden world that exists beneath a veil or cloud. God suddenly withdraws, revealing the world below (Matt, 2009). This world can refer to different things, but here I consider that it may also stand for an unconscious world, a world that exists in a different psychic dimension from the conscious one that we usually apprehend.

An effort to study an intrusion occurring in the physical world was carried out by the English physicist, David Deutch (1997). Deutch noticed the presence of shadows within some laboratory procedures that he believed could not be accounted for by the factors present in these experimental contexts. He then designed an experiment, using a single source of coherent light (such as a laser) that he projected in a completely blackened out room. He studied from different positions and angles how the light then appeared. He discovered that, in addition to all of the possible ways the beam of light could manifest itself, there still remained a shadow that seemed to come from out of nowhere. Deutch concluded that this shadow could only be emanating from a parallel universe.

Apropos of the title of this chapter, and from a linguistic standpoint (at least in the English language), I see the word, *nowhere*, as being conjoined through having the same spelling with the expression, *now-here*. Furthermore, I have come to think that there is a kind of experiential connectedness between *nowhereness* and *now-hereness* that is analogous to Einstein's concept of space-time as being a single dimension. This suggests that in undergoing the experience of *nowhereness*, in which one feels lost within the immediate surround, one may be in a literal state of *now-hereness* as well. However, the possible sense and vital presence that the experience of *now-hereness* affords is frequently lost, as one—in order to avoid the pain and disorientation of feeling lost in the world—often clings to familiar reference points. Despite its implication of affirming one's presence in the world, *now-hereness* may, in an abstract sense, also refer to the experience of the joining of pure time and space, or of what we may consider to be, *nowness* and *hereness*. Furthermore, the abstract form of this experience may leave one unable to experience, one's '*isness*,' or one's own personal existence or being. Similarly, when impersonalized, *nowhereness* can also be seen as *no-whereness*, and conjure up the experience of not knowing if there is even a *where* where one could be. These ideas will be developed throughout this chapter.

A common psychoanalytic belief is that we are unable to get beyond our own subjectivity, that much—if not all—perception is interpretation (Greenberg, 1981). I believe that within unconscious experience there is no experiencing subject and no separate object that is being experienced. These two have merged along with the context in which such experience occurs. Therefore, unconscious experience would appear to exist beyond our subjectivity and may appear to us simply as a reality, yet a reality in which our presence or actions are experienced of a piece with what is happening. Furthermore, the separate experience of one's own self may not be able to occur consciously. The philosophers of the Self have averred that the experiencing eye—or perhaps the 'I'—cannot experience itself in the act of the present event of seeing (Organ, 1968). Such experience may exist alongside of, or in a separate experiential dimension from, perspectivistic, subjectively based, and intersubjective conscious reality. In that reality, all or most perception is thought of as interpretive and relative. Perhaps unconscious experience may then be present in awareness, although not consciously so. Furthermore, there would be no room for personally generated distortion in unconscious experience: there is, once again, no longer the presence of a possible distorting subject and no separate object to be distorted.

Of great importance to the 'present inquiry'—a favorite term of Wolstein's—is Einstein's discovery that time and space are relative to one another. They are, according to Einstein, not separate dimensions. Rather, there is a single space-time continuum that exists in addition to their nominal dimensional separateness. To be in the dimension of space is also to be in the dimension of time and vice versa. As Freud has said that the unconscious is timeless, the present may be considered timeless as well, since—in psychic life—there is always a timeless present without which the past and future would have nothing to stand in relation to.

The Italian physicist Carlo Rovelli (2017) claims that existence in the subatomic quantum world of infinitesimally small phenomena is relational and interactive. He asserts that things come into existence only because they are interactively related to other things. Thus, consciousness, having an experiential source and a separate object of this experience, is such an interaction and, therefore, apprehends 'reality.' It can also be said that past and future are conscious of the present, but the present—like a quantum wave that can stand alone—may be understood to be unconscious of them.

Since there is a gap between an experiencing subject and what she or he is experiencing, time, however minute the amount, would be required to experientially traverse this distance. The structure of consciousness and the act of being conscious may then be considered to create not only the reality of the dimension of time, but of the world as well. If we understand conscious experience to be conscious of what is outside of itself, then this same perspective might imply that each conscious act would also extend one's world and, thereby, might further even create the very world that consciousness could then be conscious of, a possibility that will be later discussed in the section on quantum physics. However, unconscious experience—like the present tense—would not apprehend any such temporal interval. Nor would the world be stretched or extended by it since what in conscious experience would be apprehended as relative and—as a separate subject and object—would be experienced as already complete. An additional issue is the scope or dimensionality of what we might think of as the integral wholeness of unconscious experience, which might (depending upon the context) range from something very limited, to being as vast as the universe itself. Thus, physicists believe that the background radiation from the Big Bang (an event that occurred 13.8 billion years ago and took over 13 billion years to reach us, traveling at the speed of light, i.e., 186,000 miles per second), is still in our consciously experiential space-time present. The present may facetiously be said to be out of the dimension of time, but then it may never have had to be 'in time' to begin with, since the present—by definition—is already when events are happening. As we all originally derive from the Big Bang, and later by way of the substance of the stars, such substance may be present for us in some inchoate way as unconscious experience. This is alongside of the conscious observations and determinations that we can make about this gigantic cosmic event. Thus, the 'snow' we once saw on our television screens before the first programs of the day aired is thought by physicists to actually be a manifestation of background or microwave radiation from the Big Bang (Rosenblum and Kuttner, 2011).

Similar considerations apply to space. Since space exists between objects, consciousness would be required to experience these separate contextual aspects. Unconsciousness, because of its merged quality, would in a strict sense be unable to do this. So, when Freud said that the unconscious is timeless, he might have added that it is spaceless as well. This implies that the analytic concept of psychic space—and of course, movement within such space—can only take place consciously, thus subject to the structure that the consciously conceived laws of physics would impose, a condition crucial to ideas presented later in this chapter. In contrast, undergoing the experience of doing something as we are doing it, to be entirely in the present without awareness of ourselves as subject or to any objectified aspect of self, is to be undergoing unconscious experience.

Such was my own experience many years ago while climbing a high sand dune on a trip to the Sahara Desert in Morocco. Looking around when finally reaching the top, I suddenly felt bewildered, as I was faced by what was, for me, a featureless landscape that seemed to go on forever. I said, almost as though talking into the air (although in the presence of a companion who was now on top of the dune as well), that I felt I was in the middle of nowhere. She coyly replied, "Nowhere is spelled now-here." Hence, the title of this chapter.

My initial conscious experience of a clear separation between myself and the dune as I approached it gradually gave way to a growing sense of my being an extension of the dune. I gradually became less aware of the dune and also of my own person as the one negotiating the climb. The dune became increasingly experienced by me to be as much a part of me as I was of it, as though we were becoming experientially one. This comes close to what I imagine as being unconscious experience: a kind of union between myself and the sand dune, which did not include a clear cognizance of my separate personal being, nor a knowing awareness of the surround. Here we have an example of a process of initially conscious experience gradually transforming into unconscious experience, as the awareness of self and otherness fades. This stands in sharp contrast to later illustrations of how unconscious experience may suddenly appear, seemingly from out of nowhere.

My feeling of bewilderment at the dune at least affirmed my presence—albeit uncomfortably so—with my later ascension into full consciousness, expedited by my comment and my companion's mind-expanding reply. This part of the experience brings to mind what Heidegger (1949) wrote about the experience of dread. He said that dread appears when everything that is familiar falls away from us, revealing nothing. Dread, he chillingly writes, reveals nothing! Since consciousness implies an aware relationship between self and an outside world (i.e., from a psychodynamic point of view occurring around personally problematic issues), unconscious may be to be literally *un-conscious*, which is to say, to remove traces of our own consciously problematic involvement in these issues. Here, one is '*unconscious*' to what has been conscious experience (Wilner, 1999). Furthermore, as Rovelli (2017) has emphasized, in the quantum world—which I think applies to the unconscious realm—things do not exist as isolated entities. They first come into being and may continue to exist because of their interactive relationship to other things. What this may mean is that unconscious experience and 'the unconscious' may be constituted of dynamic and now merged relational events that are going on 'presently,' which is to say timelessly, 'within it,' rather than constituted, e.g., primarily of fixed, separate, and isolated feelings, memories, and wishes. Furthermore, as an expression of its relational nature, what may be present unconsciously would again include the now merged contexts in which these events take place. This appears to give unconscious experience a paradoxically dual nature. In having nothing that is external to it—like a particle in the particle/wave duality in physics—it seems uniquely singular, and, linguistically, best expressed through nouns. Yet, like the wave, it also has a kinetic and dynamic multifaceted relational aspect, which may be best conveyed by verb.

The merged nature of unconscious experience also loosely corresponds, both in my view and now on a cosmic scale, to what in physics might also be understood to be a singularity, or points of absolute density. Examples are the original globule of gas or matter of the Big Bang, the great density and gravitational pull of small neutron stars that were created out of gigantic stars that have collapsed, and the absolute gravitational force that is thought to exist at the bottom of black holes. Such experience might manifest itself consciously, for example, as the apprehension of single waves or patterns and, analogously and psychically as our experience of the condensations of primary process. The physicist David Bohm (2002) might think of this phenomenon and experiential event as the singularities of the dynamic unconscious having become enfolded within consciousness.

Einstein discovered through his monumental general theory of relativity that space curves. It curves as a function of the gravitational pull of the mass of the bodies of matter that occupy it. According to Rovelli's (2017) reading of Einstein, these bodies do not simply exist in space, they constitute space and are also a result of space itself curving around them. Einstein used the image of a cosmic mollusk that is curving its now granular surface, the stuff that Einstein said space is made of, around the gravitationally strong masses of bodies that are near them. These are fascinating ideas. For instead of space being a vast nothingness, it was thought of by Einstein to actually be constituted of this granular substance. Rovelli (ibid.) takes this even further by averring that, in the quantum world there is—in fact—no such thing as nothing. This notion echoes Freud's assertion that negation and, by extension, nothingness, does not exist in the unconscious. The seeming nothingness of space may be thought of in an analogous psychic way as being constituted out of the possible substance of unconscious experience awaiting conscious realization. Hence, Heidegger's (1949) formulation of dread as revealing nothing might only be the conscious awareness of this unconscious presence.

What may be thought of as the strong gravitational pull of a significant psychic issue, i.e., its 'gravitas,' may now be considered to curve psychic space as well. It might even enclose what may be a problematically generative issue to the point that a consciously separate experiencing self and a correspondingly distinctive consciously experienced object may merge. Such self and object may even become consciously reversed due to the possible proximity and juxtaposition of these originally separate objects now occupying a kind of psychical curve together. Juxtapositions such as these may actually be possible, since—as Wolfson, (2003) has said—the curvature of space-time from the perspective of relativity theory can be infinitely sharp (p. 235). Such an enclosure might ultimately create a sort of psychic black hole or metaphoric unconsciousness in which relational unconscious psychic events would be able to continue within this shield, or under this Kabalistic cloud or veil, play themselves out. Similar to a black hole, it would suck new proximal conscious experience into itself. At times, the conscious experience of this might be a weird anthropomorphic mix of a seeming boundary-permeable and surrealistic nature, which I think might be the basis for actual surrealistic artistic expressions. Creative individuals who appear to be in such a state, those whose experience—like the unconscious itself—seems opaque to us, may present as aberrant extremes: psychotic, autistic, immersed in a drug induced state, or simply dreaming. Though he was referring to the quantum world, the title of Rovelli's (2017) book *Reality Is Not What It Seems* is quite fitting in this context to our inquiry.

Similarly, Einstein showed through his Special Theory of Relativity (1905, as described by Rovelli, ibid.) that time and space are not what we ordinarily think them to be either. He demonstrated that they were not independent entities that existed 'out there' and were not the same all of the time and everywhere. He showed, for example, that time moved faster due to the weaker gravitational pull at higher altitudes than at lower ones. His work also generated the oft-repeated example of how someone could hypothetically travel through time. He proved that a space traveler in a rocket ship that is approaching the speed of light may, upon returning to the Earth, have aged little. But the people who remained on Earth would have aged, perhaps, generations. The traveler would, in effect, be journeying into the future in relation to those that she or he had left behind. We may speculate that from the perspective of unconscious experience, the traveler in the rocket ship may not appear to have aged in relation to an outside observer because this traveler has, in effect, been unconscious: the traveler has largely been outside of time and space and, therefore, can be aware of nothing outside, as there is no externality. As nothing can travel faster than the speed of light, we might further wonder that if one were to hypothetically travel at the speed of light, might there be nothing outside to be conscious of? The traveler inside the ship might simply become an unconsciously experiencing event. Everything would instead be experienced to be of a piece, a psychic oneness (Wilner, 1980). Furthermore, and in a loosely analogous way, the traveler's experience might be considered a kind of singularity that, here, would experientially draw everything close to itself as with a black hole while being experienced to be part of nothing else. Since no light from such a hypothetical light speed or even near such light speed event can reach an outside distant observer at the instant at which the event occurs, it may be said to be—as Einstein termed it—in the "observer's elsewhere," (Wolfson, 2003), as B. Budick (personal communication) points out, i.e, unable to be consciously experienced. Furthermore, from a vastly different perspective than the one which an observer might have, time and space may seem to have been jumbled: an effect may appear to have actually preceded what, to a first observer, would be seen as its cause.

Unconscious experience may also be thought of as being analogous to the hypothetical and mysterious dark matter in space. This is matter whose existence is inferred through its ability to exert a gravitational force by bending space, and is believed by physicists to constitute about 25% of space's matter (Rovelli, 2017). Dark matter has never been seen, though new detectors have been built and new experiments performed that show promise in more directly proving its existence.

The eminent physicist, Stephen Hawking (1988), who studied the subject of black holes extensively, points out that things don't just enter black holes, something also comes out. This is in the form of radiation and heat that tell physicists a great deal about the nature, origin, and possible fate of these extraordinary cosmic structures. I think the same thing can be said about our relationship to unconscious experience. The unconscious may, in a sense, be said to suck in conscious experience (e.g., my separate sense of self, and that of the outside sand dune). But how does anything emerge from it? We know about dreams, slips of the tongue, the parapraxes of everyday life. We need only wait. But how might unconscious experience be explored, if possible, more directly?

Consider now the work of Werner Heisenberg (1962). His uncertainty or indeterminacy principle states that one cannot, for example, determine the location of an electron in space and its momentum at the same time, as the act of measuring one of these dimensions affects and renders indeterminate the measurement of the other. In other words, the attempt to determine something about this subatomic particle, to consciously try to pin it down, causes other dimensions of this same particle to behave chaotically. Similarly, as Lacan (Wilden, 1973) has said, the signifier can never fully encompass what is being signified. Here, this can be understood as due to what is being signified increasing and shifting in a quantum sense as a result of a signifier being formulated in order to try to encompass it. This idea will be explicated in both a quantum way and through the application of Heisenberg's uncertainty principle to clinical work below.

The effect of this principle can be illustrated through the example of what happens when one attempts to enclose an electron in a smaller and smaller space. The velocity of the electron increases as a result, as though it were trying to escape from the tightening enclosure. What is striking here is that while the electron is rushing about, with only a probabilistic but no definite location that one can observe or determine, it is said to perhaps even cease to exist. The implication here is that it is the electron's interaction with an observer that creates its existence, without which it is thought not to be real. Transposed to the unseen contents of the unconscious, such contents may be said to truly be nowhere. Furthermore, Heisenberg suggests to us by extension that the very act of directly trying to make the unconscious conscious, a hallowed goal of psychoanalytic practice, may be like a cat trying to chase its own tail to actually create more unconscious flux.

The analytic space: *The Adventures of Tom and Jerry*

In everyday clinical work, we usually arrive at some understanding about what a patient may be doing or feeling, or we may interpret what we think are the unconscious determinants for these experiences. Believing that we have actually figured out what is going on and why—and not simply continuing to process, associate to, or analyze it—affects the way that we and the patient will experience things and behave with one another. Like the mouse who warily eyes the actions of the cat without making it too obvious that it is doing so, the patient may sense the point at which the analyst may be about to come in for a deterministic kill. If the analyst is simply continuing to think it over and/or associate to it, no determination (thus no creation of indeterminacy) would take place. But once the analyst tries to actually pin down or make real what may be going on in the patient's unconscious, the entire clinical context may shift.

How then to make an interpretation if consciously focusing on the target of the interpretation not only shifts its location, but may change the total gestalt. This would, at the very least, seem to make whatever interpretation that was to be made less efficacious. For example, if the cat eyeing the mouse was a researcher who needed the mouse to be a subject in an experiment, little purpose would be served if the mouse, now in a state of panic, chewed off one of its own feet as a result of perceiving the now analytic cat trying to interpretively trap it.

Analysts have long stated that a good interpretation makes itself. From the present perspective, the analyst would not be trying through her or his actual person to make the interpretation. Rather, it would seem to be happening on its own, unconsciously, we might say, as part of the flow of the process and as a contextual event.

But what if the analyst is bent on actually making the interpretation? Psychoanalysis is, after all, not behavior therapy. Patient and analyst not only check each other's behavior, they also read and sense one another's feelings and tension levels, which then affects the entire experiential field. Patient and analyst may then regulate each other in such a way that the analyst is then not so zealous about making the interpretation. Yet, what if this does not happen? One possibility is that the analyst may deterministically shift the focus from interpreting something to the patient, to trying to restrain her- or himself from wanting to interpret or actually not do so. The problem would now be that this new deterministic intention would continue to create indeterminacy and uncertainty, but in a different way. The analyst might be left wanting to be certain about something without creating further new uncertainty. Old habits tend to linger. The analyst may abhor the experience of feeling that she or he is getting nowhere: she or he may also be experiencing now-hereness in a de-realizing and de-personalizing way, as well. Interestingly, the clinical context has now shifted from trying to make a determination (the erstwhile interpretive desire in order to avoid uncertainty), to now living in the midst of it. As with Einstein's mollusk, which he described as closing in on what it increasingly surrounds (Rovelli, 2017), the analyst is increasingly enclosed in a psychic space. She or he has metaphorically become a now trapped cat or, from a Stephen Hawking perspective, is inside a black hole. This analyst is being pulled down by the gravitational force of her or his own interpretive desire, which may have altered, as Wolfson (2003) might say—the geometry of psychic space-time.

A number of different things may happen at this point. The analyst may become less controlling and allow things to play themselves out as they will, while simultaneously trying to stand outside of the situation in order to observe (a la Levenson, 1972) the unfolding of the clinical pattern in its many homologous and isomorphically transformative ways. The problem here is that the analyst is now metaphorically also inside of the black hole and not just standing outside of it. Standing outside would have enabled the analyst to be in a position to more objectively observe possible emerging patterns, although in the quantum world it appears to be possible to be in two different places at once (Rosenblum and Kuttner, 2011). People on hallucinogenic trips who experience themselves to be standing on a shelf in a room looking down on themselves sitting on the floor may well know this phenomenon. Just speaking, the analyst may act as a kind of smoke signal to the patient, who may rush in to rescue the analyst by saying anything. This, alone, might be sufficient to call the analyst back to consciousness by breaking the psychical gravitational pull. But the patient may also offer a more focused resonant response as well—much as my sand dune companion did with me—that might release the analyst from her or his Heideggerian dread, a true interpersonal intervention.

An additional possibility at this point is that the analyst can take advantage (not intentionally, of course!) of this trapped position and realize that she or he can become more attuned to, even fascinated by, her or his own more unconscious emanations (such as associations, fantasies, and possibly the awareness of sudden physical sensations and where they might lead) in the spirit of William James' scioustic, or self-moving experience (1890).

A final possibility I consider in this situation is that the analyst may come to realize that her or his experience of no-whereness and impersonal, and unreal now-hereness, may also be a kind of experiential window or door that can open up on to startlingly different kinds of experiences, like, for example, the Kabalistic revelation.

I will now offer a clinical vignette that illustrates some of the surprising possibilities and directions that what I think of as unconsciously generated clinical experience can take.

Some years ago, I was seeing a young woman in analysis who, during one session, was crying so incessantly and profusely that I became distressed. Nothing I was able to say or do was able to stem the flow of her tears, which I wanted to do—at the very least in order to make myself feel better. I was, during this particular session, also uncomfortably aware of feeling physical discomfort, and a vague general bodily feeling of being tugged. I was also dimly aware during this time that she was pulling tissue after tissue from my tissue box in order to wipe away her tears. As I think of it now, the tissues might have represented discrete packets of quanta, the stuff of the quantum world. She suddenly said, "I'm using up half of your tissues." I unreflectively then replied, "I think you're using up half of my *issues*." Amazingly, the crying suddenly stopped. We then were able to talk about why she was so upset, as well as how my issues may have intruded into the treatment, and how they might be implicated in why she was feeling the way she was at the time. What began as a discussion of issues turned at this point into a more associative interaction, although—unlike her crying—not profusely so. An outside person observing this interaction might well wonder who was the analyst and who was the patient? Here, I think that both of us were both.

This case illustrates one way in which underlying unconscious experience—in terms of a reversibility of subject–object, a possible merger between the two, and a kind of anthropomorphically surreal feeling–can manifest themselves in clinical work. My physical feeling of being pulled at in the context of what the patient said was so vivid that I didn't think I was simply being pulled at 'as though' I were the tissues in the box. Instead, I came close to actually experiencing myself (as if in a borderline or psychotic state, or as a merger of consciousness and unconsciousness) as almost being—not simply the tissues, but what now seemed like more sentient objects can, as context and subject/object in the quantum world—become one. In my view, this is a stronger illustration of emergent unconscious experience than the example of the sand dune. Rather than a blending of experience of self and dune, the above example felt decidedly crazy, as I experienced myself as not only one of the pulled tissues in the box, but as if the tissues had suddenly become me.

Dudley Young, in his book *Origin of the Sacred* (1991), said that "to the medieval mind, language words, are not used simply in order to refer to something else. They are also thought to be able to summon up the very powers they name" (p. xxvi). Words are constitutive of these powers in the same way that objects in space also constitute space itself. The words and those uttering them may then merge with these powers in what is akin to being in an unconscious state. This perspective has some interesting and amusing implications when applied to some of the issues in this chapter.

One of the implications is that in the presence of a psychical gravitational pull, the words and expressions that may come to one's mind may themselves be instances of the contextually bounded pull itself, with what is said also being an expression of it. One is no longer, as in human consciousness, solely saying or thinking something about something else. Instead, the act of speaking or thinking is, as Young (1991) implies, also what is actually happening, i.e., the kinetic aspect of unconscious experience. In fact, one may not even be able to avoid this. The metaphoric curvature of psychic space may be placing the words and the issue that is doing the gravitational pulling together, where the words themselves may now generate their own gravitational pull—much as Heisenberg might think of as the effects of deterministic actions. In the later more focused section on quantum mechanics, this convergence of words and issues might be referred to as entanglements.

When it comes to the medium of words and language, what—in the previous case—might seem to be an example of a somatically tinged delusional experience may appear to be more of a thought disorder, with an attribution of reality to the concrete hearing of words.

Thus, the expression, 'something is the matter.' Psychodynamically, we literally think that for there to be an issue in the treatment, or for the patient to enter analysis to begin with, something must be wrong. This is also phonetically and concretely heard, in line with Rovelli's (2017) assertion about the interactive relational nature of being, as also being "sumthing," the possible sum of a number of different things must be wrong. Thinking about Einstein's theory about how heavy bodies in space have considerable mass as part of their matter, enabling them to curve space, led me to conjoin the connectedness, if not also the actual sameness, between the physical and psychical realms. To me, this suggests that things that metaphorically are matter, that are the matter, as well as do matter, curve psychic space.

This line of reasoning may hint at alchemy, a subject of great interest to Jung (1959), for it suggests the possibility that the act of unconsciousing, and perhaps also that of consciousing may be able to turn the psychical and physical into one another. In this scenario, the consciously physical shows up psychically as unconsciously generated experience while the unconscious psychical appears in the conscious physical world. This is also a subject of intense and controversial interest in the area of quantum mechanics (as I will soon consider), as to whether conscious observation is what causes objects to exist in the objective physical world to begin with. The possibility of unconscious experience appearing in the physical realm has been expressed through Jung's psychological rule, which states that when a portion of the psyche is split off, the world must embody and enact this submerged or cut off part. In other words, psychic substance does not simply disappear. According to David Bohm (2002), it may continue to exist physically, would be in the world's implicate order, and might be—in the eyes of psychoanalysts for example—seen as psychosomatic manifestations.

For example, considering that perhaps it was actually not me that was generating the experience of the word—something as the sum of things and ruling out for the moment the possibility that I was being controlled, as David Deutch (1997) might consider, by some alien power from a parallel universe—the words 'not me' are a prototaxic expression of how I, as an interpersonally trained psychoanalyst, actually think, thus further explicating the theme of this inquiry. In interpersonal parlance, the expression 'not me' (now heard as a noun) refers to what Sullivan referred to as prototaxic experience, the Sullivanian equivalent of the Freudian unconscious. So, in disavowing personal conscious involvement in what had come to my mind, as I did, I would wind up inadvertently affirming it (from a different trajectory) as possibly emanating from my own unconscious. I may have been saying, in effect, that it was my own 'not me,' my own unconscious, that was coming up with these words and expressions and not, for example, a separate contextual field.

As I was writing this, I began to feel overwhelmed with meaningfully sounding associations and no longer wanted to experience any more, which—like my patient's tears—felt as though they could keep rolling in, much like copies of the broom that kept rushing out along with the flood of water in "The Sorcerer's Apprentice" portion of Disney's *Fantasia* (1940). This began to feel as though I might be starting to fall into the grips of a mollusk myself or was metaphorically nearing a black hole that was now threatening to draw me in. I found myself thinking, "no more!, no more associations." I was then chagrined to realize that I was now hearing these words as also contradicting what had just been my conscious intention; instead, now saying, "no, don't stop, I want more," as in, "no! no!, more! more!"

At this point, I gave up, though apparently not entirely so, for I also heard the word "I" in the expression, I give up, in the way Wolstein (1974b) sometimes referred to it. He said that the 'I' is first-person singular and is the part of one's self that is most directly connected to unconscious experience. My surrender was apparently then complete, and I experienced no further associations or hearings that were themselves instances, that is, actual happenings of the very issues I was exploring. That is, except for one, which may be the most significant of all.

No hands to no mouth

After now reaching what I thought was the point of completion of this essay, I realized that I had left out another example. Ironically, it was one I had thought about for years and was so much a part of my thinking that it had probably slipped my conscious mind as possibly being the core expression of the emergence of linguistic unconscious experience. It simply is the expression of something coming to mind as both referring to and being itself an instance of this something literally inserting itself in my awareness and thereby objecting to, that is, 'minding' the way I was now seeing and understanding things. Whatever came to mind then provided some corrective to the way I had first apprehended whatever the context was. This suggests that there may be a pull within gravitationally influenced contexts toward unconscious experience as a means of resolving problematic and open issues. Since unconscious experience, in having nothing that is external to it, is structurally already whole, therefore, in its oneness, it's a model for what resolution itself actually is.

In the terms of Gregory Bateson's (1979) logical rule—which a scholarly colleague (R. Eichler, personal communication, 2017) informed me actually comes from Maimonides—the named cannot, without committing a logical error, also be the thing named. I realized that I was then in runaway and flagrant violation of this rule. But I then laughed to myself when I realized that this rule held only in relation to conscious experience, in which subject and object are separate from one another. In other words, from an unconscious perspective, one may be in violation of an unconscious logical rule by not expressing or perceiving things in such a way that they are instances of what one is consciously referring to. The caveat here is that the rule would apply only when one is actually in the midst of a psychical gravitational pull. This is actually a tautology. For in the throes of such a pull, one may not be able to do otherwise to begin with, just as outside of such a pull, one would not be able to unconsciously, if you will, live out the instances of what one is referring to as they would not be of a piece.

I, therefore, distinguish unconscious experience from the psychoanalytic concept of enactment. In enactment, as in conscious experience, one is enacting something from a different place (e.g., some aspect of an interaction with another). In the living out of unconscious experience, there is no different place. One is thus not acting in a particular way because of something else. By implication, a different formulation and/or other words that may be introduced in order to get to the meaning of something would not, from this perspective, be necessary: the form is already here. It is considered to already be present and whole in the words, actions, and experiences that appear on their own in the way that they do in the immediate clinical context and in subsequent experiences. As Groddeck (1977) has said, the meaning of something is revealed by its consequences. This study of unconscious experience is not about meaning-seeking, whereby one hears, observes, or thinks about something that is thought to be significant and then pursues its possible meaning, which is often done at the expense of not following experience that appears on its own in our awareness.

Lest I leave you with the impression that being in the throes of unconscious experience is mostly strange fun and games, I want to describe an event that occurred many years ago, and was perhaps the most frightening experience I experienced up to that point in my life. I was alone in my apartment reading Kafka's *Metamorphosis* (1952), which—as I think of it now—may have symbolically depicted what Kafka may have been going through as he was writing it. The telephone rang, and I went into a panic. For at that very instant, I underwent the experience of having no hands with which to lift the receiver, no mouth from which to speak into it, and, perhaps, though I did not know for sure, no voice to be able to utter any words. I, in effect, had experientially become the beetle that Gregor Samsa had turned into in the book. This experience, no doubt, speaks to the fragility of boundaries and, of course, my own, between consciousness and unconsciousness, the physical and psychic worlds, reality and unreality, and sanity and insanity. Unaware of how immersed I had become in the book, I didn't simply merge with it (since a merger between two separate entities should contain or manifest aspects of both) or, if I did, the book was stronger. In any event, it took me over, and the beetle in the book experientially became me.

I consider now that I had, so to speak, crossed the line in the way that I did because the buffer or alarm system that shocks us into realizing that we are getting too close to the psychic vortex was missing. Unlike at the sand dune, and in my distress with my patient, I had no experience here of nowhereness first. I had no chance to experience any unconsciously generated emanations, and fell directly, if you will, into a psychic black hole. The creature in the book, the beetle, like the unconscious, could not directly come out; in the book, Samsa did hide his beetleness behind a living room couch. In addition, like another literary creation of Kafka's (1952), a hungry black panther that replaced a starving man as an exhibition in a circus cage, the unconscious may be conjectured to be able to find full release only by taking over or experientially becoming those who get too close to it. This might be a further expression of unconscious experience allowing nothing to be external to it (i.e., the starving man was no longer present in the story once the panther appeared). As psychoanalysts, we know better than most how metaphorically hungry unconscious experience can be, making its presence felt in our conscious world.

The felt realness of such experience can be frightening or as it was for me, terrifying. Sullivan (Levenson, 1996)—possibly prompted by his spider dream in which he experienced a giant spider about to devour him and from which he woke in terror—is known to have said that clarity is the last thing one experiences before becoming schizophrenic. Furthermore, this same clarity does not hint at the unfamiliarity of nowhereness that comes with the experience of dread. Instead, and quite to the contrary, one recognizes the reality in such an experience all too well, and can feel—as Sullivan did—almost consumed by it. For example, a psychotic person may have the delusion that he or she is Jesus, yet this might be understandable: the person has the belief that he or she is Jesus because the real person as her or his own self has vanished from awareness. Immersed in working on this chapter as I have been, I may not even have been aware of my own personal absence. Has it actually then been me who has written it? A rigorous quantum perspective might leave this as an open question or—as Rosenblum and Kuttner (2011) would put it—an enigma. Let us beware of overexciting the mollusk.

There is a precedent, by the way, in pop culture for a Being taking over a man and then becoming him. It is not from *Invasion of the Body Snatchers* (Finney, 1955), but rather from the 1931 novel *The Shadow Laughs* by Maxwell Grant (Deutch's shadow, we see, has returned in another form). In this story, a dark supernaturally appearing (male) figure called The Shadow manifests himself as a large shadow in a room and makes himself invisible by hypnotically rendering others unable to see him, invading the home of the wealthy society figure Lamont Cranston in order to take over not only Cranston's identity but his corporal being as well. The Shadow is a crime-fighting figure who wants to use Cranston's person and position in order to work more effectively toward his purpose. The real Cranston then disappears. What is relevant here is that in the 30 to 40 years or more that the character appeared in various media, The Shadow was known as Lamont Cranston, wearing the disguise of the strange figure of The Shadow, rather than the way it originally was: The Shadow now appearing in the form of Cranston, who had vanished.

So, may the unconscious have once intruded into the reality of conscious life in such a way that we may no longer appear or perhaps even know or remember how we originally were? Or, is it consciousness that is the intruder? Like the chilling words that were part of the introduction to each Shadow (Jung's term for the unconscious) radio program, "Who knows what evil lurks in the hearts of men? The Shadow knows," suggesting that unconscious experience, despite Heisenberg, may actually be able to know.

In his book *The Origin of Consciousness in the Breakdown of the Bicameral Mind*, Julian Jaynes (1977) holds with consciousness as being the original intruder. In his textual analysis of early Greek writings, Jaynes observed from pauses that occurred when the action shifted or when a character changed direction in behavior or thought, that these shifts did not occur because the character was now thinking in a different way. Jaynes concluded that these characters were experiencing auditory hallucinations in the form of the gods telling them what to do instead. Such hallucinations might seem to us to be an expression of unconscious experience although, to the early Greeks, they may have been reality, events that were happening in the world.

The extreme nature of this example might rule out for us that the gods' speaking was actually happening, but it does open up the issue that with our present reductive psychoanalytic emphasis on subjective experience, and perception as interpretation, how can we know what reality—even an objectively indeterminate one—may actually be? Without this knowledge, does our sense of conviction in our actions and beliefs falter as a result?

In his book *The Hidden Reality*, Brian Greene (2011) considers eight different scenarios of the multiverse, a generic term for parallel universes. One version seems particularly relevant here. It is that what we take for reality is actually the result of a computer-driven program from a parallel universe. Notwithstanding the difficulty in distinguishing unconscious experience from reality, it raises the additional question of whether reality itself is, so to speak, for real. Furthermore—instead of what we take to be reality being a computer-driven program from a parallel universe—might we also consider it to be a projection from the timeless and spaceless events going on in our own unconscious psyches? Does this then raise the question that parallel universes and unconscious psyche might be one?

It is, perhaps, ironic that in undertaking to explore the possible existence and nature of unconscious experience, we may have lost our hold on reality in the process, a possible Heisenbergian phenomenon. But perhaps reality may simply be inside a black hole where it becomes infused with unconscious experience, awaiting its reemergence as reality once more, its shadowy veil now lifted yet now as a reality deeply connected with unconscious experience we may have at once personally lived. As Wolstein (personal communication, 1975) often put it, not just once personally lived, but also suffered and endured. This might constitute an additional merger, or perhaps under the right psychical gravitational conditions, a possible connectedness, now between reality and unconscious experience.

Entanglements

Just as Rovelli (2017) introduces the concept of quantum gravity to bring together Einstein's general theory of relativity (which applies to large stable bodies) and quantum mechanics (which pertains primarily in experimental procedures and contexts to the ever-changing flux of subatomic particles), I have used the concept of unconscious experience to try to bridge the apparent gap between the physical world of reality and the psychical realm.

I now see the conjoined terms of nowhere and now-here as a kind of Rosetta Stone or code that can vivify for us the immanence of unconscious experience. If, as Rovelli (2017) asserts, within a strong gravitational field objects do not simply move through cosmically voluminous entities such as space and time, but rather also become part of their fabric, then experiencing nowhereness may be to be experiencing profound truth. Namely, that this experience, this event, can only be of now-hereness as well, as there is in such merged contexts in which object and space/time have become one, no other space and time, so to speak, to be in: that there are at these instants no space except here, and no time except now. Some physicists (Greene, 2011) have claimed that the creation of each new such reality constitutes a new parallel universe.

I have tried here to discuss two forms of unconscious experience. I think of the experience of the sand dune, the experience of being pulled at with my patient, and that of the beetle as being totalistic, in that there appeared to be nothing in my awareness that was finally external to these experiences, including a sense of my own separate self. In contrast, there are the largely verbal emanations that I assume originate from unconscious experience, in which one is aware of oneself, but one's experience may at times feel as though it is being taken over from without, here possibly from a different dimension. An exception to this is the case of the protagonist of *Time and Again* (Finney, 1970/1995) Simon Morley, who—while being in the 1880s instead of in his own time of the 1970s—was able to retain consciousness of himself and of his own world. As analysts in clinical work who may be undergoing manifestations of our own unconscious experience, we naturally hope to retain this. However, should we, at moments, lose our sense of ourselves, as well as that of time and space, we similarly hope that they will return, appearing as they perhaps might from seemingly out of nowhere.

In their book *Quantum Enigma* (2011), Rosenblum and Kuttner present different enigmas (some alluded to above) posed by work in quantum mechanics that appear relevant to the present conception of unconscious experience. The authors refer to these phenomena as enigmas largely because they defy our sense of reality. In one experiment, a pair of photons or electrons were made to interact and then sent off in opposite directions at such a distance from one another that not even at the speed of light would they be able to communicate or affect one another within the frame of the experiment. Astonishingly, they were still found to be mysteriously linked to each other, in that an effect introduced to one was found to show up in the other, thus apparently violating the basic law of physics that states that nothing is capable of exceeding the speed of light. Quantum physicists have coined the term 'entanglements' to refer to the effect of having the two particles interact with one another with such a later effect.

Physicists whose theoretical base is more in relativity rather than in quantum theory might account for the possibility of such a phenomenon—generally described as Bell's Theorem—as being due to the bending of space through gravitational pull or by space, like a gigantic organism squeezing itself so that such a connectedness might be possible. However, from a psychical perspective of unconscious functioning, these links and entanglements may be occurring in other-dimensional and possible parallel universe contexts that may be hard to even conceive of; things that would, within the space-time continuum, otherwise be consciously experienced as being separate and perhaps unrelated to one another. The string theorist Lisa Randall (2005) addresses the issue of other dimensionality by positing the existence of 13 rather than five dimensions in nature—eight of them microscopic or sub-microscopic and hidden—that originally included the dimension of time.

Psychoanalytically, I have thought of the possibility of other dimensionality in a practical sense, as existing only in certain psychodynamically generative contexts, or contexts in which there are open issues 'pulling' for resolution. But this may be too limited a perspective. Thus, quantum physicists who at first restricted their conceptions, such as entanglement, to subatomic particles and under tight experimental conditions now consider that their theories may hold for the macroscopic world as well—this being despite that they were formerly thought to be the exclusive province of Newtonian classical theory and Einstein's relativity theories. Similarly, introducing some of these conceptions in physics—in terms of a larger psychophysical world—has extended my view of unconscious experience in ways that I could not have first imagined. Nor, as we shall see, could my vision encompass the utterly strange nature of reality as unveiled by the field of quantum mechanics.

Other quantum enigmas that appear relevant to the present study are the result of experiments that appear to show that something may be in two different places at the same time, and the related enigma of experiments that suggest that the physical world may not actually exist independently of and prior to observations made of it (Rosenblum and Kuttner, 2011). While the full details of these experiments lie beyond the scope of this chapter, some of the ideas upon which they are based may be briefly mentioned as they pertain to the present concept of unconscious experience.

A central idea is that subatomic particles have a wave function in addition to their physical reality (Rovelli, 2017), analogous to how we might think unconscious experience may be the wave function of conscious thought and observation. This wave function can spread beyond the location that an object is thought to be, placing it in what is termed a superposition state, whereby parts of it are considered to exist in two places at once: they can be observed experimentally, for example, to be in two different boxes that are separated from one another (Rosenblum and Kuttner, 2011). Unconsciously, we would consider this to be an experientially indeterminate state, a state in which something could manifest itself consciously as two different realities. The above experiment has led to a further enigma.

According to Neils Bohr's Copenhagen interpretation (Rovelli, 2017) of this experiment, the particle is not assumed to be physically present in a box until it is consciously observed, which is then said to collapse its wave function. A variation on this experiment concerns how this experiment is set up to begin with. One here may look into one of the above two boxes and see a complete atom in one of the boxes. However, we cannot say in which box the atom will appear. Or, one may begin by looking into the same two boxes and see parts of the same atom in both boxes instead. In other words, the physical world is not assumed to exist here in the same way that it is later being observed. Quantum scientists say that the past of these objects is also, in effect, changed in order to produce the different outcomes we later find. Rosenblum and Kuttner (2011) add that we can choose how we will observe things, but not the particular outcome we will encounter.

Numerous experiments have failed to conclusively refute these strange findings regarding the subatomic world. Attempts have also been made to replicate one of the above experiments, but without a conscious observer (Rosenblum and Kuttner, 2011). If, for example, the two box experiment is set up with a Geiger counter determining whether an object is physically present in a box rather than a conscious observer, this Geiger counter is said to fall into a superposition state because of its own possible entanglement with the particle: it may be found to appear to be both firing and not firing at the same time, tantamount to something being there and not there at once. Thus, the presence of entanglement, whether it be with a human observer or a Geiger counter keeps quantum scientists from being able to prove conclusively that the physical world exists independently of observation and measurement, human or otherwise. In other words, as perhaps with the present conception of unconscious experience, there is no such outside, independent, or real existence.

In the context of this chapter, the apparent connectedness or perhaps correspondence between different verbal expressions—such as with things coming to mind—can be thought of as due to the presence of a psychic wave. It can also be due to what we might consider to be an original entanglement that encompasses both noun and verb. There is thus a figurative reference to an independent reality and the separate concrete action of coming upon it, the same expression now being in a state of superposition that allows it to have reference in these two different ways at the same time. The first reference would, again, be about the consciousness of what this expression refers to, corresponding to the way we might perceive the real world to be. The latter refers to the experience of being in the actual unconscious act, (the concrete act of what the expression consciously refers to being lived out and actually happening in the world), e.g., of its 'coming' to mind, or the awareness of my own 'not me.' Because these events often happen so quickly, seemingly from out of nowhere, we ordinarily do not experience them as being part of the conscious and stable reality of the world. Rather, we may think about them instead as something like the result of the intrusiveness of the unconscious. The nature of the unconscious may be such that, as anthropologist Levi Strauss (1962) said, the primitive mind does not allow anything to be alien to it. Like a singularity of maximum density in the physical world, unconsciousness would, for example, have the capability of having both actions, the kinetic aspect of the unconscious and figurative references of the above expressions merged within itself in a superposition state. Thus, unconsciousness would also not allow anything to be alien to it. Unconscious merger may itself then be a kind of superposition state.

Physicists, such as Rovelli (2017), again try to reconcile what appears to be a basic incompatibility between quantum and relativity theories through trying to develop a theory of quantum gravity. We might say that there is a similar psychoanalytic schism between a more consciously oriented relational orientation. In this concept, there is a keen interest in what is outside of oneself, including intersubjectivity and a separate concept of psychic agency, and what may be considered to be a more holistic and integrally unconscious-oriented approach in which emergent experience would be thought to be capable of appearing as and from an already constituted and originally present whole, a kind of unconscious universe. This may be what unconscious experience may originally present to us prior to our consciously creating a picture of reality from it.

This presents an interesting issue. If, as according to one segment of quantum thinking, participation via the acts of a conscious observer may be necessary to collapse a wave function and have things experienced as real for us, then the apparent inability of consciousness to perceive unconsciousness naturally renders the unconscious dimension finally and essentially consciously invisible and apparently unreal to us. As with Heisenberg's aforementioned electron, we might then say only that the unconscious may tend to exist. Yet, like dark matter, and even more so, dark energy, which is said to constitute about 70% of the energy in the universe (Rosenblum and Kuttner, 2011), along with anti-matter (all in the physical realm), unconscious experience may be as correspondingly dominant in the psychical realm. Again, it is now-here, but yet seemingly and paradoxically nowhere to our conscious minds and experience of reality at the same time. It thus seems to be the concrete act of observation that creates the reality of the object. What we take from our conscious assumptions about what reality is places the form of this object in our view. But it is the act of concretely observing it that makes the experience of it real, that is, actually there for us in the world.

The Lone Ranger as the unconscious?

But what might be the view of reality that unconscious emergence ultimately places before us? Speculation from cosmologists and spiritual thinkers point to an intrinsic meaningfulness and connectedness in both the psychic and physical universes, an extraordinary and integral kind of wholeness that William Blake summed up in his poem *The Auguries of Innocence* (Blake, 1803; Gilchrist, 2017) by saying that the whole world may be seen in a grain of sand. Yet, there is another thought now from the quantum world that suggests that this apparent connectedness may finally all be random, although Rosenblum and Kuttner (2011) offer a strong statistically based argument that this is a highly unlikely possibility. Perhaps then, the answer may rest ultimately with what we believe. As Wolstein (1974a) has said from the psychoanalytic perspective of unique experience, each person must create her or his own interpretation and philosophy of her or his own life, and one's own understanding of the world.

We may now see that when Wolstein wrote that unconscious experience is private and not shareable, this includes with and from one's own self as well. Going back to the earlier citation from the philosophers of the self, the experiencing eye or, psychically now, the 'I', cannot experience itself in the act of seeing. What may be in the unconscious, this reservoir of psychophysical being, we cannot see directly, like trying to look inside a black hole without getting sucked in: in fact, we are already of it. We may only be able to speculate and infer what, to use a spatial metaphor, may be inside of it as is our wont. But we may be able to be sensitive and receptive to its emergence, its often apparent intrusiveness. We may be able to sense its incredible and singular contextual connectedness and meaningfulness. Thus, instead of an object appearing to be in two different places at once, perhaps it is we who create the reality of there being two different places to begin with, with the object then appearing to follow suit. Like Wolfson's (2003) comment about how gravity is the geometry of space-time, not only our outside 'real' contexts, but those of our personal contextual dispositions of mind may coalesce with one another and create, like the interpretation that seems to make itself, what will finally and consciously emerge for us as ourselves and the world. As such emergence is action-in-context, an event that both creates and is the world, it is likely we can both 'unconscious' our experience and expose the oftentimes incredible weirdness and omnipresence to our conscious eye of the possibilities of the geometry of space-time as well. Thus, not only can an object, such as a subatomic particle be in two places at once, but in a grand entanglement of superposition, the two places may also be the same place.

Perhaps, Rovelli's (2017) sought-after theory of quantum gravity can provide a window onto the kinds of geometries, the strange configurations, that could allow for entanglements and linkages that could defy the basic laws of what nature can allow. If gravity is, as Wolfson (2003) implies, also geometry, then not only are we speaking about gravitational forces operative within space-time, but of the entire macroscopic universe being in a state of perpetual quantum-like flux with ongoing gravitational-like pushes and pulls. For physicists like Rovelli (ibid.) who seek, through a theory of quantum gravity, a link between the macroscopic and subatomic worlds, Wolfson's comment appears to offer a direction.

I never expected in beginning this exploration of unconscious experience to stumble into, like falling into a rabbit hole, some of the weird ideas and phenomena of the physical world, especially as developed in the field of quantum mechanics. I began by seeking to explore or trying to find a correspondence between the psychical and physical domains, only at the end to find, as Rosenblum and Kuttner (2011) so clearly articulate, that these two dimensions may be inseparable from one another. That is, without a conscious observer to observe it, there may be no world. And, furthermore, without unconscious experience to apprehend both it and observer as one to fuse our experience of them into an integral whole, we might not be able to even be part of a world that we may have through our observation created.

So, does unconscious experience actually exist? Is it Real? As a process of emergence into awareness as with the sand dune and the crying patient examples, it appears to exist and be real. At least, a conscious observer might label or 'realize' this to be unconscious experience. I refer to this in a paper (2005) entitled "The Lone Ranger as a Metaphor for the Psychoanalytic Movement from Conscious to Unconscious Experience." The Lone Ranger, as he rode off at the end of one of his adventures, never said who he was and never sought thanks or reward. However, by his keen observations and actions, he, like perhaps unconscious experience, was a brief, but powerfully impactful presence in the contexts he affected, although never identified with those contexts. Paradoxically, and again like unconscious experience, his presence was inseparable from his subsequent disappearance. Like a quantum enigma, he seemed to be there and yet not there in reality at the same time. He never appeared to have a self beyond the actions he undertook. Even his mask, which at first suggested another identity in the world, finally just masked the fact that he may have actually been hiding nothing, may have had nothing to hide. He left the people he had helped always asking and wondering, "Who was that masked man?" Or here, who or what was that unconscious intrusion that seemed to come from out of nowhere? Someone would then usually say, "that was the Lone Ranger." But then no one really knew—before the story of his origin was created for him after the first four or five years of the character's existence—what a Lone Ranger was or, as we ask here, what is unconscious experience?

Like my view of unconscious experience as primordial, perhaps like a psychical version and offshoot of the Big Bang itself, the Lone Ranger first appeared as a radio program character in early 1933. But he stood out from other fictional hero characters by being the only such figure to not also have another real identity in the world (at least then) that could mask, deflect from, or add to who or what he was. As we can only speculate and theorize about what unconscious experience is, we can ask—once again—if it actually is? The Lone Ranger could only at first be the Lone Ranger. He could not be self-conscious as he had no separate self originally present to be conscious of. But even if, hypothetically, he did have a conscious separate self, it would be at once merged and integral with everything that he was and the context he was now part of. As with unconscious experience, 'Lone Rangerness' could only exist for us as a reality in the world at the instant of our observing consciousness and enduring experience of this Lone Ranger's presence.

A key question here is, what makes for an enduring experience? An experience can endure unconsciously through a strong pull or entanglement or a personally problematic one as well, which puts one in a position to be taken over by it. If, as I have tried to illustrate, this can happen vis-a-vis a sand dune, a box of tissues, and, most powerfully, a novelistic creation of a beetle, why not then, the experience of a fictional character such as the Lone Ranger as well? Of course, from the position taken in this chapter about unconscious experience and merger, this could only occur if the Lone Ranger, like unconscious experience, also became, in part, oneself as well.

Note

1 This is an expanded version of a paper presented at the William Alanson White Institute on December 1, 2017.

References

Bateson, G. (1979). *Mind and nature*. New York, NY: Dutton.
Blake, W. (2019). *Auguries of innocence and other lyric poems*. Scott's Valley, CA: Create Space Publishing.
Bohm, D. (2002). *Wholeness and the implicate order*. New York, NY: Routledge.
Deutch, D. (1997). *The fabric of reality*. New York, NY: Penguin.
Disney, W. (Producer), & Grant, J., & Heumer, G (Writers). (1940). *Fantasia* [Motion Picture]. United States: Walt Disney Productions.
Finch, H. L. (1977). *Wittgenstein: The later philosophy*. Atlantic Highlands, NJ: Humanities Press.
Finney, J. (1955). *Invasion of the body snatchers*. New York, NY: Dell.
Finney, J. (1970/1995). *Time and again*. New York, NY: Scribner.
Gilchrist, A. (2017). *The life of William Blake*. Mineola: Dover Press.
Grant, M. (1931). *The shadow laughs*. New York, NY: Street and Smith.
Greenberg, J. (1981). Prescription or description: Therapeutic action of psychoanalysis. *Contemporary Psychoanalysis, 17*, 239–257.
Greene, B. (2011). *The hidden reality*. New York, NY: First Vintage Books.
Groddeck, G. (1977). *The meaning of illness*. New York, NY: International Universities Press.
Hawking, S. (1988). *A brief history of time*. New York, NY: Bantam Books.
Heidegger, M. (1949). *Existence and being*. Chicago, IL: Gateway.
Heisenberg, W. (1962). *Physics and philosophy: The revolution in modern science*. New York, NY: Harper & Row.
James, W. (1890). *Principles of psychology*. New York, NY: Dover, (1950).
Jaynes, J. (1977). *The origin of consciousness in the breakdown of the bicameral mind*. Boston, MA: Houghton-Mifflin.
Jung, C. (1959). *AION*. Princeton, NJ: Princeton University Press.
Kafka, F. (1952). *Selected short stories: Metamorphosis, 19–90; A hunger artist, 188–201*. New York, NY: Modern Library.

Levenson, E. A. (1972). *The fallacy of understanding*. New York, NY: Basic Books.

Levenson, E. A. (1996). Aspects of self-revelation and self-disclosure. *Contemporary Psychoanalysis*, *32*, 237–248.

Levi Strauss, C. (1962). *The savage mind*. Chicago, IL: The University of Chicago Press.

Matt, D. C. (2009). *The essential Kabbalah: The heart of Jewish mysticism*. New York, NY: Harper One.

Organ, T. (1968). The self as discovery and creation in Western and Indian philosophy, In P. T. Raju & A. Castell (Eds.), *East-west studies on the problem of the self* (pp. 163–176). The Hague, NL: Martinus Nyhoff.

Randall, L. (2005). *Warped passages: Unravelling the mysteries of the universe's hidden dimensions*. New York, NY: Harper.

Rosenblum, B., & Kuttner, F. (2011). *Quantum enigma*. Oxford, UK: Oxford University Press.

Rovelli, C. (2017). *Reality is not what it seems*. New York, NY: Riverhead Books.

Wilden, A. (1973). On Lacan: Psychoanalysis, language and communication. *Contemporary Psychoanalysis*, *9*, 443–470.

Wilner, W. (1980). Psychic oneness: A treatment approach, In G. Epstein (Ed.), *Studies in non-deterministic psychology* (pp. 155–179). New York, NY: Human Sciences Press.

Wilner, W. (1999). The un-consciousing of awareness in psychoanalytic therapy. *Contemporary Psychoanalysis*, *35*, 617–668.

Wilner, W. (2005). The Lone Ranger as a metaphor for the psychoanalytic movement from conscious to unconscious experience. *Psychoanalytic Review*, *92*, 759–776.

Wolfson, R. (2003). *Simply Einstein*. New York, NY: W.W. Norton.

Wolstein, B. (1974a). Individuality and identity. *Contemporary Psychoanalysis*, *10*, 1–14.

Wolstein, B. (1974b). "I" processes and "Me" patterns. *Contemporary Psychoanalysis*, *10*, 347–358.

Wolstein, B. (1982). The psychoanalytic theory of unconscious psychic experience. *Contemporary Psychoanalysis*, *18*, 412–437.

Young, D. (1991). *Origins of the sacred*. New York, NY: St. Martin's Press.

EISTEIN'S ELSEWHERE: DISCUSSION OF WILNER

Burton Budick

Warren sees the unconscious as residing in Nowhere. For a physicist familiar with Einstein's theory of special relativity, Warren's Nowhere has remarkable similarities with Einstein's Elsewhere.

Some background.

Time is normally described as divided into past, present, and future. If we plot time on a vertical axis, then the x (or horizontal) axis is the present, negative values of x (values below the x axis) are in the past, and positive values of x refer to the future (Figure 1.1).

In relativity Einstein taught us that we need to speak of events. To specify an event we need two coordinates, an x or spatial coordinate to specify where along the x axis the event occurred, and t, a time coordinate to specify when the event occurred. That is the case because <u>where</u> an event occurs depends on <u>when</u> it occurred, and vice versa. In relativity we have

Time:

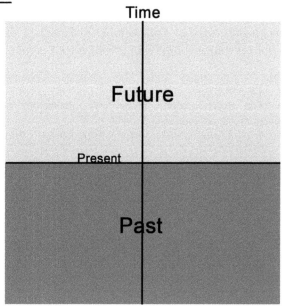

Figure 1.1 Time

to speak of space-time rather than time and space (positions) independently. We will see the practical application of these ideas shortly.

In special relativity, past, present, and future are represented as in
Figure 1.2. We will label the points on the vertical time axis in years, and
on the horizontal x axis in light-years. A light-year is the distance light
travels in one year, approximately 100 trillion miles.

Suppose event A is in the present. We locate event A at the origin. For
event B to be in event A's future it must lie in the cone specified by the
two 45 degree lines. Event A has time to send a light signal to influence or
change event B. That is because the distance from A to B is less than the distance that light can travel in the time interval that separates A from B. There
is time for someone at even A to send information to change the outcome at
even B. Another way to state this is that B and A are causally related.

Suppose that we look at events A and C. The distance between them is
three light years, but the time between is one year. A light signal emanating from A cannot reach event C in one year. A and C are not causally

Spacetime:

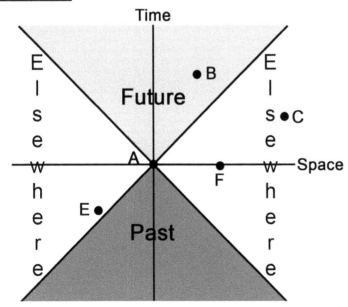

Figure 1.2 Spacetime

related. Even C is in event A's Elsewhere. Elsewhere occupies as much area as past, present, and future combined. In fact, it is not possible to be certain of the time sequence of the two events. By that I mean that an observer moving close to the speed of light might see event C happening before event A. A second observer moving at a different speed or in a different direction might see event A preceding event C. To a third observer the two events might be simultaneous.

Now let the events be occurrences in two dreams being related by a patient. An oft repeated remark on the part of the patient might be, "But the events in the first dream had to precede the actions in the second dream, but they couldn't have." The observer, in this case who might be the analyst, remarks that events in dreams are not related by causality. We can't be certain of the time sequence between occurrences in the Unconscious. For me this is the salient point in Warren's paper. The dreams come from Nowhere.

Chapter 2

Into the frog swamp

Jungian conceptions of the unconscious in practice

Michael Monhart

I thank the White Institute for the invitation to speak about the Jungian conception of the unconscious as part of their yearlong colloquium series. Along with my gratitude, I commend their willingness and curiosity in inviting speakers from a wide range of psychoanalytic theories. It is a move that I hope other institutes emulate.

I also welcomed the opportunity because of the emphasis on the unconscious.

I regard Freud and Jung and other psychoanalysts of their time as, in a sense, early cartographers, drawing maps of a new territory, discovered partly through their patients, and to a large degree, based on their own journeys, their own self-analyses. Today we might look at these early maps and say some territories are too small, or too large, or wonder about what was included on the map, the areas that early mapmakers would assign to a dragon. That is why I think this book is so important—it at once takes us back to our roots of working with the unconscious and allows us all to compare maps, and through dialog, gain shared knowledge of this inner world.

Though I very much appreciated the opportunity to submit a chapter to this book, then as I thought about it more, I questioned my sanity. Jung was a prolific writer of essays, books, and letters. The *Collected Works* total 20 volumes. The Philemon Foundation is currently publishing additional material with approximately 16 volumes published or in process. The Foundation references 35,000 as yet unpublished letters. So, there is a mass of written material, of which a large portion is still unpublished. Jung wrote over a long span of years. He presented his medical dissertation in 1902 and he continued writing until his death in 1961.

In such an enormous corpus of work, and with Jung's wide-ranging interests in fields outside of psychology, along with a writing style that can be rambling and digressive, one can find not only contradictions but also just about enough evidence to contend that Jung said just about anything! Despite this profusion of words, one finds cryptic insights that, read today, seem to presage many developments in contemporary psychoanalytic theory. Given the broad range and immense amount of his writings, I can't hope to cover every aspect of his theory, nor do I want to make this chapter too theory heavy. I'm going to instead try and lift out some of his ideas that I have found clinically useful and let them resonate with you who may have very different theoretical backgrounds.

One of the problems reading Jung is the tension between his self-professed stance as an empiricist, reporting only observable facts and, on the other hand, language that some find overly mystical, metaphysical, or epistemologically suspect. This tension explodes in complexity in his alchemical works where one can be left dazed and confused, longing for some grounding in psychological clinical description. We have problems then not only with the amount of material but also with its varied manner of presentation. Either sticking to empirical data derived from word association tests or launching into the seemingly contradictory abstruse language of alchemy would probably leave you more bored.

Initially, following the title of one of the key volumes of his *Collected Works*, Vol. 8, *The Structure and Dynamics of the Psyche*, I planned a two-part chapter. The first part would be a grand tour of the structure: persona, ego, Self, personal and collective unconscious, archetypes, followed by case material. I believe that Jung started with structure but ended with dynamics and that one of the reasons he went off into alchemy was to try and find a model of psychic dynamics. But following such a plan would have been too lengthy, so I am going to start with the presentation of case material and then look at some of the imaginative experiences and images contained in Jung's *The Red Book*. In 1913, Jung, through active imagination, began his self-exploration of the unconscious. *The Red Book* is his record of these experiences, expressed in narrative and handcrafted images. As I go along, I will try to elucidate particular Jungian ways of conducting analysis and working with the unconscious.

When I mentioned to a friend and colleague at the Jungian Psychoanalytic Association in New York City my burgeoning anxiety about this chapter, he suggested I start with what attracted me to Jung in the first place. I first encountered Jung as a 19-year-old living in a Trappist Catholic monastery. Strange perhaps for a 19-year-old boy, I thought there was more to this unconscious business than sex! Seriously, though it was actually some of the monks who introduced me to Jung, finding in him someone who they believed was sympathetic to religion while at the same time providing a method to help them with psychological issues. They encouraged me to start writing down and thinking about my dreams. In dreams I sensed a movement within me, but beyond me, I found images that were multi-valent, confusing, illuminating, inspiring, and critical. Primarily, I found a telos, a forward orientation that seemed to say that if you work on the dreams, then they develop and that changes your sense of self.

Jung referred to this sense of telos, of forward orientation, as individuation. The Jungian analyst Murray Stein has written

> The theme of individuation sounds through Jung's writings, like a leit-motiv, from the time of his break with Freud onward without pause to his death. All things considered, it is perhaps his major psychological idea, a sort of backbone for the rest of the corpus.
>
> (Stein, 2006, 196–197)

The concept of individuation will serve as a backbone to the material I will present. For Jung, individuation was a possible goal beyond symptom relief and an analysis of the repressed contents of the personal unconscious. Jung emphasizes, however, that individuation is not individualism. In his essay on individuation, he describes the process:

> But the more we become conscious of ourselves through self-knowledge, and act accordingly, the more the layer of the personal unconscious that is superimposed on the collective unconscious will be diminished. In this way, there arises a consciousness, which is no longer imprisoned in the petty, oversensitive, personal world of the ego, but participates freely in the wider world of objective interests. This widened consciousness is no longer that touchy, egotistical bundle of personal wishes, fears, hopes, and ambitions which always has to be compensated or corrected by unconscious counter-tendencies; instead, it is a function of relationship to the world of objects, bringing the individual into absolute, binding, and indissoluble communion with the world at large. The complications arising at this stage are no

longer egotistic wish-conflicts, but difficulties that concern others as much as oneself.

(*CW* 7, 1966: 275)

In the analytic process the developmental traumas along with the multiple superimposed projections of the repressed personal unconscious are worked through. Yet, there is also always a listening to what can be emerging, where is the territory where the personal problem touches upon the "communion with the world at large" (*CW* 7, 1966: 275). One analogy for the listening process is listening to a piece of classical music for example, where one listens, registers, retains the memory of what has come before, what themes or colors of orchestration have been played, while at the same time listening forward, listening for the perhaps subtle changes as a theme is developed.

The concept of individuation and listening to the forward edge of a dream or of clinical material is the orientation of my presentation of, first, some case material and secondly, an excerpt from Jung's *The Red Book*. In both the case material and in Jung's *The Red Book* experiences, we can see glimpses of the individuation process in play, a movement from the personal to the collective. As I noted, I want to spare you all the grand tour of trying to rush through each and every one of Jung's theoretical conceptions of the psychoanalytic process, so in these capsules of case and *The Red Book* experience, I will focus in particular on the idea of the complex, on what I regard as specific features of Jungian dream interpretation, and on looking for the archetypal level of an image. Let's start with the clinical story.

Case presentation

The analysand is a man in his mid 20s. I have been seeing him for three years, once a week. He has been very regular in attendance, missing only a few sessions in that time for a vacation. In the very first session, noting that he only had come because his sister had been pestering him to do so for months, he said, "Resistance is the theme of my life. My main intention or goal, if one can have one, is to overcome resistance." He described wanting to learn computer programming, but said he wastes time playing video games, hanging out on Internet forums, reading but not really reading. He felt like he has to move forward, that people say "you're young" but he feels stuck, and he brought up the image of a crossroads. In one of the first sessions he said, "Is it laziness that I just have to overcome? But working 9:00 to 17:00 is insanity." He described the laziness as a demon that just comes up. I asked, "Like two or three hours go by and then one asks what happened?" To which he replied, "Yes, that's it."

In just this first session, even in these few lines of dialog, a stage is set which I'd like you to keep in mind: resistance, a desire to overcome resistance but also an underlying question—if 'working 09:00 to 17:00 is insanity'?

In the second session, he started talking a little about his family and, to his surprise, was quite moved. He is mostly estranged from his mother. His parents divorced when he was quite young and he went to live with his father as he entered high school. Later in our work he talked about being bullied in elementary school, of his mother over-reacting to the point that he no longer talked about it with her.

Most of the sessions in the first months revolved around the issue of resistance/laziness and talking about the relationship he had with his mother. As our work went along, he had less and less contact with her; the fixation and grip of what I will call the maternal complex lessened; he got work with a start-up company and has stayed there these past years, working long hours and being given increased responsibility and higher positions.

In the first month, he had these two dreams:

The first:
I am in car with my father and sister. We're driving along next to a beach and the ocean. There are some waves. We go up a steep incline, like along a cliff. Reach a plateau and a flat area. There's a small shack there, selling lobsters. They're pre-cooked, ready to eat. We eat.

The second:
I am walking through a huge mansion; it's dark, empty and eerie. It's not a nightmare just very suspenseful. There are no hallways, just rooms connected by doors. In all the rooms there is a faint light. They are minimally furnished, a bed, maybe a night table. Maybe my grand-mother lived in this house. There's one room with a lamp, like a bea-con, but not enough light. On a lower level a room with a sink. There is a weirdness, creepiness to the room with a light because it also had a closed door. There is a door to the basement, which is properly lit. I

opened the door to the basement and went downstairs. It is safe, normally furnished, lit, more normal and home-like.

I look at dreams that occur early into the analytic process, as generally, though certainly not always, as an important diagnostic and prognostic tool. Often, they can depict the 'state of affairs' in the conscious and unconscious; they give the lay of the land so to speak. They can also have some predictive capacity, or some suggestions of how to proceed at first. I say predictive not in the sense of prophetic but more as a proposal of the work that can be accomplished. I would actually expand this notion of initial dreams to include anecdotal/descriptive material that is recounted in the early sessions. In an essay on dream analysis Jung wrote about dreams at the beginning of the process, what are sometimes called "initial dreams" in Jungian terminology. Jung writes,

> It frequently happens at the very beginning of the treatment that a dream will reveal to the doctor, in broad perspective, the whole programme of the unconscious. But for practical reasons it may be quite impossible to make clear to the patient the deeper meaning of the dream.
>
> (*CW* 16, 1966: 343)

I don't want to be too Jungian in my style, but I will make a short digression. Jung, in a 1934 letter to James Kirsch wrote, "As soon as some patients come to me for treatment, the type of dream changes. In the deepest sense we all dream not out of ourselves but out of what lies between us and the other" (Lammers, 2016, p. 62). There can be a number of factors at work here perhaps—the initiation of analysis sparking images from the unconscious, or perhaps, that there is a relationality that quickly ensues between the analyst and patient both consciously and unconsciously (which is why Jungian patients dream Jungian dreams and Freudian patients dream Freudian dreams?). Kirsch himself suggests that it shows the intersubjective, relational aspects in Jung's approach to the analytic process, and I think it is an indication of Jung's acknowledgment of the essential relationality of the analytic process.

In the case of my analysand, he had not previously paid much attention to dreams, and subsequent to these dreams, he only reported a handful. He had no real associations to any of the images in these two dreams. I do think, however, that they did reveal a pathway for our analytic work together. I use the past sense 'did' here because, quite honestly, I offer a mostly retrospective interpretation that fits with how the analytic process actually unfolded.

The first dream was the most puzzling. There were no associations whatsoever, nor any suggestions as to the setting. I noted at the time, to myself, the location. We were not in the ocean; while there are waves in the sea, we were not in the toiling midst of waves of unconscious affect. In that respect, it reflects the state of affairs, a current condition. Yet the ocean, as a symbol of the matrix of the unconscious is there, adjacent, in view. The mother is not there. There is a steep incline that leads to a plateau where pre-cooked lobsters are being sold in a small shack. In fact, in the first six months or so we took a steep incline as he separated from the affective grip of a negative maternal complex. In time we got to a plateau, higher up the cliff, where he gained perspective, moved into his own apartment, and commenced working. The lobsters are still a bit of a mystery, but one possible interpretation is a transferential implication in that part of the relationship that did emerge was a mentor–mentee dynamic where, in a sense, I took a much more advice-giving, or 'pre-cooked,' approach than I generally would. Another intriguing angle on the lobsters that was not apparent at the time of the dream was his Jewish background. Lobster as shellfish are prohibited by Jewish scriptures. For Jung, contents arising from the unconscious that offer an expansion of ego consciousness can often be perceived as transgressive, as a threat to the established ego position. Lobsters are also a food that began as a very cheap, common item but then evolved into more of a luxury. There is a bivalency here of something cheap, not valued that becomes its opposite. I'll explain in a moment why I am sticking so close to the images presented in the dreams.

The second dream gave another depiction of a 'state of affairs,' an image of how things are for him at the time. The overall description, couched in words like "dark, eerie, weirdness, creepiness," gives the impression of a haunted house. And indeed, as more personal history emerged, there was evidence of intergenerational trauma in both sides of the family. One of the most noticeable aspects of the mansion above the basement is the lack of corridors. The rooms just open one into another, with no interconnecting hallways, no liminal spaces of transition. This was one of his most persistent symptoms. When he started therapy, he had great difficulty getting out of the house, instead staying in his room, playing video games and spending time on Internet forums. He wanted to study, to learn, to develop skills but was stuck, spending hours watching a movie, playing a game, only to 'awake' and then go back to what he had started studying. If one regards the basement in the dream as the unconscious, it is where he feels normal, at home. Here again, the work over the first year or so was a movement from the safe, womb-like, unconscious affective world of video games and movies and to a move upstairs, into a world of ego consciousness and self-agency, a job, an apartment. The move upstairs, so to speak, also meant starting to develop corridors, hallways, liminal linking spaces between rooms of job, relationship, and the search for an answer to the question—is working 9:00 to17:00 insanity?

I regarded "the theme of my life is resistance," closely tied to procrastination, as a complex. For Jung the psyche, and I use that word here to encompass both conscious and unconscious, is fundamentally dissociated. While there is a central ego, in reality its place as central can be easily displaced. Yet, Jung also posits the concept of the Self as a wholeness that encompasses ego and unconscious, a wholeness that is emblematic of healing, a broader consciousness and fuller engagement with the world. The Jungian analyst Sherry Salman captures this tension between dissociation and unity, writing,

> For Jung the psyche was inherently dissociative, with complexes and archetypal tendencies functioning autonomously as multiple fields of experience. Following William James, the dream of totality that emerged for Jung was one of multiple complexes and personalities working to create wholeness, in the same sense that mysterious or distressing symptoms are usually both the wound and the beginning of the cure, because they are expressing what is pushing to be integrated into the personality.
>
> (Salman, 2013, p. 111)

We'll return to symptom being both the wound and the beginning of the cure when I talk further about the case material, but for now, let us look in more depth into the idea of 'complex.'

What is a complex? Jung asks and answers the question like this in a 1934 article:

> It is the image of a certain psychic situation, which is strongly accentuated emotionally and is, moreover, incompatible with the habitual

attitude of consciousness. This image has a powerful inner coherence, it has its own wholeness and, in addition, a relatively high degree of autonomy, so that it is subject to the control of the conscious mind to only a limited extent, and therefore behaves like an animated foreign body in the sphere of consciousness.

(Jung *CW* 8, 1969: 201)

A complex then is characterized by strong emotion and by an incompatibility with the habitual conscious attitude to such a degree that it can act like a foreign body. In practice—think of situations that seem to constellate within you a sudden mood, a feeling that I am not myself, or why in the world am I reacting in this way to this person or event, or how did I ever forget this or that or suddenly lose my temper? One image that I use is of a magnet, attracting all shards within its radius, making each shard completely part of the magnet. Then the emotion dissipates, the air clears and you ask, "What just happened?" as you return to a habitual attitude of consciousness. You can see this dynamic in the difficulty my analysand had initially of getting lost for hours in a video game or Internet forum, only to 'awake.'

Jung, in the same article, calls complexes "splinter psyches" and describes the causality:

> The aetiology of their origin is frequently so-called trauma, an emotional shock or some such thing, that splits off a bit of the psyche. Certainly, one of the commonest causes is a moral conflict, which ultimately derives from the apparent impossibility of affirming the whole of one's nature.
>
> (Jung, *CW* 8, 1969: 204)

These I think are two remarkably insightful sentences; note the etiology of trauma or emotional shock but also the causality of not being able to affirm the whole of one's nature. A complex can be caused by trauma or emotional shock but also has an archetypal core around which it clusters. In this case, the core can be seen in one of the initial comments my analysand made, "Is it laziness that I just have to overcome? But working 09:00 to 17:00 is insanity." Working with the complex involves what we can call 'circumambulating the complex,' talking through the triggers and ways the complex becomes such an "animated foreign body" with the goal of loosening its affective grip on the person. Secondly, one asks what is the root of the complex? In the first sentence of Jung's quote, we see a reference to my analysand's struggle to overcome a developmentally caused retreat into a safe, known space, a resistance to leaving the room. But the second sentence points less to resistance and more to what Jung described as an "impossibility of affirming the whole of one's nature" and to what I regard as the archetypal core of the complex. The core dilemma emerged in a couple of vignettes. In one he described a particularly difficult period in college that was precipitated by readings that made him question on a very personal, but very deep level the nature and value of the work one does in society. In another session we listened together to a comedy broadcast where the host at once humorously and seriously asked the caller to think of waking up one day, growing older in a job he didn't like and a place he didn't want to live. From this we came to a perspective that recognized traumatic aspects of his upbringing but also, at the same time, asked of the future—what would meaningful work look like for him?

In contemplating the dreams and in trying to tease out the cause and the core of the complex around resistance and laziness, I tried to adhere to what I see as one of the key aspects of the Jungian approach to the unconscious, that being, as James Hillman said, "Stick to the image." In a lecture on dream analysis Jung said the patient

> begins by associating in accordance with a theory, that is, they try to understand and interpret, and they nearly always get stuck. Like the doctor, they want to get behind the dream at once in the false belief that the dream is a mere façade concealing the true meaning. But the so-called façade of most houses is by no means a fake or a deceptive distortion; on the contrary, it follows the plan of the building and often betrays the interior arrangement. The "manifest" dream-picture is the dream itself and contains the whole meaning of the dream. When I find sugar in the urine, it is sugar and not just a façade for albumen.... To understand the dream's meaning I must stick as close as possible to the dream images.
>
> (Jung, *CW* 16, 1966: 319)

Staying close to the image, be it in a dream, a story told in a session, or in an enactment, privileges the analysand's process; it respects the psychodynamics of their conscious/unconscious balance or imbalance. It provides another standpoint to the analyst/analysand relationship, and it facilitates the drive toward telos, toward an individuation that is particular to that analysand, by giving attention and energy to the images that come from them. I have come to wonder if this sticking to and privileging the analysand's images is, in fact, a form of analytic love.

Recently, my analysand decided to take extended time away from work and go on a trip abroad, wandering from country to country. We asked: was this resistance to settling further into his work and into the sometimes messy work relationships that were part of his job? Or was this a search, a quest for a career, a way of living that was most meaningful to him? Was this trip a stage in the longer journey of his individuation? Along with the practical considerations of his current life situation, we looked at the images noted above with the readings in college and the reaction to the tragic-comic question of waking up in the future in a life not wanted. These were not images of resistance at a personal developmental level, rather they were existential questions of meaning in life. This I regard as the archetypal level of the complex around resistance and laziness, the, as Jung said about complex formation, "moral conflict, which ultimately derives from the apparent impossibility of affirming the whole of one's nature" (*CW* 8, 1969: 204). In that way, what appeared as the wound, that is, resistance and laziness, led to, if not the cure, a movement toward healing of the underlying dilemma. Once, in a session, we contemplated the mysterious ending quote of the movie *Mad Max: Fury Road*, "Where we must go, we who wander this wasteland, in search of our better selves." This seemed to be the nature of his trip and he went.

In the frog swamp: Jung's *The Red Book* experiences

This practice of staying close to the image, of fully exploring what is inherent in the image as opposed to free-associating around it, is perhaps best and most dramatically illustrated in the experiences written and painted in Jung's *The Red Book*. In some ways, one could look at *The Red Book* as Jung's wandering through a wasteland, searching for his better self. Jung begins the chapter in his autobiography titled "Confrontation with the Unconscious" (which recounts *The Red Book* years) describing the "inner uncertainty" and "disorientation" that he felt after the break with Freud (Jung, 1965, p. 170). The disorientation invoked by the separation with Freud provoked in Jung a question of what was the myth that he now lived by? (Jung, 1965, p. 171). This echo of the Mad Max character's search can be heard in the path to Jung's quest for a myth by which to live, a wandering into the desert spaces and inner solitude so vividly portrayed in *The Red Book*.

Very near the beginning of *The Red Book*, Jung wrote this passage,

> But the spirit of the depths said: "No one can or should halt sacrifice. Sacrifice is not destruction, sacrifice is the foundation stone of what is to come. Have you not had monasteries? Have not countless thousands gone into the desert? You should carry the monastery in yourself. The desert is within you. The desert calls you and draws you back, and if you were fettered to the world of this time with iron, the call of the desert would break all chains. Truly, I prepare you for solitude.
>
> (Jung, 2009, p. 123)

Sticking to the monastery, which I think is the central image here, drawing in representations of sacrifice and the call of the desert, I find a symbol for the container, the vessel of Jung's *The Red Book* encounters.

For Jung, the call of the desert was a voice to the voices, a call to the others in his inner world. This call would eventually, in a theoretical sense, be incorporated into his formulation of the prospective nature of the process of individuation. This call of the voice to the voices also brings us to the image of the monastery as a place where monks live 'alone together.' This 'alone together' is the heart of the image. The monastery is not a hermitage; it is not a solitary hut in the mountains. It is a container in which men and women live solitary lives together. I have spoken with many monks and nuns, East and West, over the past three decades, and, invariably, the difficulties of living in community comes up as a theme of conversation. Think—a monastery is where people come to live together not because they know and/or like each other but because of a common aim. It is a little like the inner world of the psyche. You are not sure who you are going to meet. You choose where you live, but not you who live with. You might like or not like your fellow monks or nuns, but you have to learn to live with them in a spirit of understanding.

In the course of the imaginations that form the *The Red Book* experiences, Jung encountered animals and people that challenged him, perplexed him, infuriated him, inspired him, all animals and people alike that were facets of himself that pressed for integration. One of these was the character of Philemon who himself emerges first out of a serpent, and then a man called Elijah. Philemon, in his final guise, was a guru-like figure for Jung. He reminisced in *Memories, Dreams, Reflections* that,

> Philemon and other figures of my fantasies brought home to me the crucial insight that there are things in the psyche which I do not produce, but which produce themselves and have their own life. Philemon represented a force which was not myself. In my fantasies I held conversations with him, and he said things which I had not consciously thought. For I observed clearly that it was he who spoke, not I. He said I treated thoughts as if I generated them myself, but in his view thoughts were like animals in the forest, or people in a room, or birds in the air, and added, "If you should see people in a room, you would not think that you had made those people, or that you were responsible for them." It was he who taught me psychic objectivity, the reality of the psyche. Through him the distinction was clarified between myself and the object of my thought. He confronted me in an objective manner, and I understood that there is something in me which can say things that I do not know and do not intend, things which may even be directed against me.
>
> (Jung, 1965: 183)

Jung's encounters with Philemon, at times insightful, at times paradoxically puzzling and bewildering, usually challenging, led him to the experience of what he called the objectivity of the psyche, that is, the inner figures who appear in dreams and in active imaginations have a distinct quality of otherness to them. They are of me and not of me. Hence, from an ego perspective, from the standpoint of my 'I' identity, they are to be related to, and carrying this further, to borrow the formulation from the French philosopher, Paul Ricoeur (1992), I find myself through relation with the other, though in this case the other is an inner other. As I mentioned earlier, these inner others can be perceived from the perspective of the ego as transgressive, as a loss to the autonomy of ego identity, but it is in the shared space of relationship, with inner others or interpersonally, with people, that a fuller sense of one's Self emerges.

Jung concludes *The Red Book* with the "Seven Sermons to the Dead." These are extended lectures by Philemon, though Jung has ample room to pose questions.

I wanted to choose a passage from these sermons, from Jung's dialogs with Philemon, but frankly, with a limited wordcount for this chapter, it is hard to quickly give any short excerpt that on the surface doesn't seem baffling or even absurd, such is the language in which Philemon speaks. For Philemon speaks in the language of the unconscious; he speaks with the seeming contradictions and reason-resistant language of dreams. In the passage I did choose, and I warn you it is a bit lengthy, Philemon first appears as a magician, then turns into himself, mirroring how dream images morph, appearing in different guises. After the excerpt of the dialog between the two, Jung attempts to sum up the lessons he has been learning. He, in a sense, is doing what we do when we take the language of the dream into an interpretation. But perhaps you'll be as much baffled by Jung's interpretation as by the actual exchange with Philemon!

> But in the fourth night I saw a strange form, a man wearing a long coat and a turban; his eyes shone cleverly and kindly like a wise doctor's. He approached me and said, "I speak to you of joy." But I answered, "You want to speak to me of joy? I bleed from the thousandfold wounds of men."
>
> He replied, "I bring healing. Women taught me this art. They know how to heal sick children. Do your wounds burn you? Healing is at hand. Give ear to good counsel and do not be incensed."
>
> I retorted, "What do you want? To tempt me? Mock me?"
>
> "What are you thinking?" he interrupted. "I bring you the bliss of paradise, the healing fire, the love of women."
>
> "Are you thinking," I asked, "of the descent into the frog swamp? The dissolution in the many, the scattering, the dismembering?"
>
> But as I spoke, the old man turned into Philemon, and I saw that he was the magician who was tempting me. But Philemon continued:
>
> "You have not yet experienced the dismembering. You should be blown apart and shredded and scattered to the winds. Men are preparing for the Last Supper with you."
>
> "What then will remain of me?"
>
> "Nothing but your shadow. You will be a river that pours forth over the lands. It seeks every valley and streams toward the depths."
>
> I asked, full of grief, "But where will my uniqueness remain?"
>
> "You will steal it from yourself," Philemon replied, "You will hold the invisible realm in trembling hands; it lowers its roots into the gray

darknesses and mysteries of the earth and sends up branches covered in leaves into the golden air."

(Jung, 2009, p. 540)

After this interchange, Jung tries to reason through the encounter, writing,

> I gathered from Philemon's words that I must remain true to love to cancel out the commingling that arises through unlived love. I understood that the commingling is a bondage that takes the place of voluntary devotion. Scattering or dismembering arises, as Philemon had taught me, from voluntary devotion. It cancels out the commingling. Through voluntary devotion I removed binding ties. Therefore, I had to remain true to love, and, devoted to it voluntarily. I suffer the dismembering and thus attain bonding with the great mother, that is, the stellar nature, liberation from bondage to men and things. If I am bound to men and things, I can neither go on with my life to its destination nor can I arrive at my very own and deepest nature. Nor can death begin in me as a new life, since I can only fear death. I must therefore remain true to love since how else can I arrive at the scattering and dissolution of bondage? How else could I experience death other than through remaining true to love and willingly accepting the pain and all the suffering? As long as I do not voluntarily devote myself to the dismembering, a part of my self secretly remains with men and things and binds me to them; and thus I must, whether I want to or not, be a part of them, mixed in with them and bound to them. Only fidelity to love and voluntary devotion to love enable this binding and mixing to be dissolved and lead back to me that part of my self that secretly lay with men and things. Only thus does the light of the star grow, only thus do I arrive at my stellar nature, at my truest and innermost self, that simply and singly is.

(Jung, 2009: 540–541)

To now ponder our way through these passages is to encounter the feebleness, the grasping at partial truths that often characterizes our encounter with the productions of the unconscious. If one sticks to the images that Jung provides, we see commingling as bondage, scattering, dismembering, dissolution through love that arises through voluntary devotion. I believe here that Jung is speaking to the nature of projection and identification, both with intra-psychic figures and in inter-psychic relationships with other people. Jung does not identify with Philemon, even though he regards him as a guru-type figure; indeed he argues, cajoles, and questions him repeatedly. Commingling is a process of bondage, of being bound to the projection onto either an intra- or inter-psychic figure. This bondage must be dismembered, and, in that dissolving, Jung proposes that he actually finds the part of his self that, in fact, does lay with men and things, in a more authentic, voluntary relationship of love. The dismembering and dissolving that Jung depicts in *The Red Book* was part of a process following the break with Freud, a period where his sense of who he was, what his own theory was, along with his role and position in the psychoanalytic movement of the time were all questioned. The catalyst for *The Red Book* experiences was a disorientation, the feeling that Jung had lost his myth, the myth that he lived by.

Heeding the call of the desert was for Jung following the call of individuation, a call very much akin to the call of vocation that monks and nuns follow into the monastery. The wound of the disorientation he experienced at this time became the source of healing as he encountered inner characters, not of his own choosing, from whom he had to at first disengage, from identification, a commingling with them, only to then recognize them objectively. This objective relationship with inner characters is what Jung refers to as the reality of the psyche.

I'll conclude with a short reflection returning to love. In his interpretation of the encounter with Philemon which we just heard, Jung says, "Only fidelity to love and voluntary devotion to love enable this binding and mixing to be dissolved and lead back to me that part of myself that secretly lay with men and things" (2009, p. 541). Love becomes the solution, in the sense of solution as the medium of the work, and also the agent of a transformation that led him back to the part of his self that, more authentically, was in relation with others.

References

Jung, C. G. (1965). *Memories, dreams, reflections*. New York: Random House.
Jung, C. G. (1966). Individuation: The function of the unconscious. In William McGuire (Ed.), *Two essays on analytical psychology, the collected works of C.G. Jung, vol. 7*. Princeton, NJ: Princeton University Press.
Jung, C. G. (1966). The practical use of dream-analysis. In William McGuire (Ed.), *The practice of psychotherapy: Essays on the psychology of the transference*

and other subjects, the collected works of C.G. Jung, vol. 16. Princeton, NJ: Princeton University Press.

Jung, C. G. (1969). A review of complex theory. In William McGuire (Ed.), *The structure and dynamics of the psyche, the collected works of C.G. Jung, vol. 8*. Princeton, NJ: Princeton University Press.

Jung, C. G. (2009). *The red book: A reader's edition*. (Sonu Shamdasani, Ed.). Philemon Series. New York, NY: W.W. Norton.

Lammers, A. C. (Ed.). (2016). *The Jung-Kirsch letters: The correspondence of C.G. Jung and James Kirsch*. London and New York, NY: Routledge.

Ricoeur, Paul. (1992). *Oneself as another*. Chicago, IL: University of Chicago Press.

Salman, Sherry. (2013). *Dreams of totality: Where we are when there's nothing at the center*. New Orleans, LA: Spring Journal.

Stein, Murray. (2006). Individuation. In R. Papadopoulos (Ed.), *The handbook of Jungian psychology: Theory, practice, and applications*. New York, NY: Routledge.

FREUD AND JUNG: SUBMISSION AND SURRENDER TO THE UNCONSCIOUS: DISCUSSION OF MONHART

Daniel Shaw

Much has been made, initially by Balint, later by Erich Fromm and more recently within the relational psychoanalytic community, of the trauma Freud caused to the psychoanalytic movement when Ferenczi was banished and shunned, ultimately because of his returning to trauma theory in his "Confusion of Tongues" paper. But now it seems that the banishing of Jung, for claiming there was more to libido than sex, was a similarly traumatic blow to psychoanalysis (and I won't even get into Adler and Rank). If we put aside the blinders and the knee-jerk contempt of the previous generations of those who dominated psychoanalysis, we may notice, for example, that Jung's concepts now appear to foreshadow today's work on trauma and dissociation, which in itself harkens back to the work of Pierre Janet, who was clearly one of Jung's important influences, and one that he did not disavow, unlike Freud. In the 21st century, can Jung's work finally receive greater respect from the so-called 'mainstream' psychoanalytic community? Michael's rich, enthusiastic chapter, first presented as a paper at the White Institute, itself only recently welcomed by that so-called mainstream, is a welcome contribution toward that end. Perhaps we are entering an era when we are not only sensitive to 'othering' when it comes to race, gender, and geopolitics, but dare I say, even when it comes to rival psychoanalytic theories! As John Lennon said, "Imagine!"

Similar to the way Michael Monhart had some exposure to Freud before turning to Jung, I had some exposure to Jung as well before my own training—mainly through the books of Joseph Campbell, which I read after finishing college in 1973. Jung's work saw a resurgence in popularity at that time, in the therapies of the human potential movement that arose with the Aquarian 'new age.' Jung had already been a significant influence in the formation of Alcoholics Anonymous. None of that—popularity, spirituality, or the 12 Steps—enhanced Jung's reputation within the religiously atheistic Freudian camp of that era.

So, maybe now is a good time for more psychoanalysts to revisit Jung with fresh eyes. Monhart gave us a Jungian feast in his chapter, but I'll only be able to pick just a few things to discuss.

Monhart's first exposure to Jung leads him to value understanding his dreams as a means of growing his sense of self. A more classically Freudian orientation might have a somewhat different focus, and would have led Monhart to wonder about what shameful sexual and aggressive, narcissistic impulses his dreams were hiding. Though those two interpretive possibilities are not necessarily mutually exclusive, right off the bat we do come upon the well-known differences between Freud and Jung. For Jung, the unconscious is a deep source of personal and human wisdom that, when accessed, provides energy and knowledge for the purpose of healing and growth, the unfolding of one's fullest human potential, and connection to the subtle and concrete energies of the universe.

For Freud, the contents of the unconscious, and their attendant conflicts, await to be released by the psychoanalyst's correct interpretations, so they can be understood and resolved. For Freud, the unanalyzed unconscious is what makes us ill; when analyzed properly with the correct understanding, better adaptation to the demands of work and love become possible.

Let me evoke Manny Ghent, in his iconic paper distinguishing surrender from submission (Ghent, 1990), to put it this way: Freud's neurotic subject is in *submission* to the unconscious, and must conquer it to be free. Jung's subject is encouraged to seek liberation through *surrender* to the unconscious. Freud fought to release himself from the grip of the unconscious, to break the code, and to thereby find the courage, through rationality and the overcoming of fear of the truth, to gain the confidence he needed to become the triumphant head of his movement. Jung believed that he emerged from his total surrender to the unconscious, the period of self-exploration that resulted in *The Red Book*, to find himself at a transcendent level of consciousness informed by the metaphysical mysteries of the universe. For Freud, Jung was a fantasist; for Jung, Freud was a reductionist. It seems that they polarized their theories to some extent due to their need to liberate themselves from and repudiate their initial dependence on each other.

Turning to Monhart's clinical material, which displays his rich, complex thinking: Monhart presents two initial dreams of his analysand. For me, they set out the patient's hope for what Michael can help him achieve. The analysand dreams that he is free of his imprisoning bond to his traumatizing mother, and that he is getting to a higher place, with a better view, without losing connection with his sister and father—without having to be entirely alone. And there they can be free and not afraid to try new things—they can even eat lobster if that's what they want. I think the patient's dream tells Michael about the kind of freedom—in Jung's term, individuation—to which he hopes their work will lead.

The second dream also, I think, lets Michael know that the analysand has been wandering and lost in spaces that seem eerie and weird, dimly lit, not really illuminated. It seems that he hopes, by going more deeply within, to find a way of feeling stable and safe. Much fascinating material emerges from Michael's far more detailed look at all the images, their accompanying associations, and the symbols from mythology that might emerge. Is there a danger in Jungian work, though, of missing the forest for the trees? The way I hear the dreams, if a simple narrative of what happens in them can be told, is that they are expressing the hope that this new relationship with Michael will lead to emancipation and freedom. The dreams are prospective in the sense that that is what actually happens in their work together.

Another point: one of the goals we recognize as therapeutic today was defined by Philip Bromberg (Bromberg, 1996) as developing the capacity with analytic patients, whatever the degree of trauma they have experienced, of "standing in the spaces" between what would otherwise be dissociated self-states. Perhaps the resonance of Bromberg's formulation with Jung's concepts popped out for you the way it did for me when Monhart quoted Sherry Salman explaining Jung:

for Jung, the psyche was inherently dissociative, with complexes and archetypal tendencies functioning autonomously as multiple fields of experience. Following William James, the dream of totality that emerged for Jung was one of multiple complexes and personalities working to create wholeness.

There's a minor amount of language there between Jung and the contemporary relational psychoanalytic concept of the multiplicity of the self and the universality of developmental trauma and dissociation. To face all the parts of the self, the bad me and not me, to recognize the fear and shame that keeps parts of self exiled, and be helped to find the courage and compassion to know the self more fully, is a contemporary relational goal, and a goal of contemporary trauma theories, much in sync with Jung's formulations.

Finally, though my mind doesn't naturally bend in the direction of the collective unconscious, I am taken with Michael's quote from Jung, where he says, and I paraphrase,

> the widened consciousness is no longer that touchy, egotistical bundle of the personal when connection is made with the collective unconscious; the complications arising at this stage are no longer egoistic wish conflicts, but difficulties that concern others as much as oneself.

That almost sounds like Jung is saying that individuation, the hoped-for outcome of Jungian analysis, is something like what I believe is the aim of relational psychoanalysis, that is, the facilitation of the greater capacity both to know oneself as a subject—self-recognition—and to be able to create and engage more meaningfully in intersubjective relatedness—mutual recognition. It may suggest as well that the Jungian analysand becomes conscious of being embedded in a socio-cultural surround that can be explored and challenged, not merely submitted to. My question for Jung, were he with us today, would be: to what extent does Jungian work value mutual recognition and intersubjective relatedness? Is that equally or less important than individuation? Like Monhart, I also had a monastic period in my life—I followed a guru in what I later came to recognize was a cultic community. At the beginning of this time in my life, I had the kind of mystical experiences that William James described in *Varieties of Religious Experience* (James, 1917), and that Jung experienced—ecstatic overwhelming experiences of cosmic awareness. Those extraordinary, uncanny experiences led me to a long exploration of the mystical, theological worlds that so fascinated Jung—and on a quest for what was being called 'self-realization.' I didn't understand then that submission and idolatry, not mutuality, was the real path in the community of which I was a member; and the outcome of my spiritual quest in this group was a kind of spiritual solipsism, not true subjectivity and certainly not intersubjective relatedness. As someone with a specialization in post-cult trauma, I have for many years seen the devastating consequences of these wrong turns toward the dark side of enlightenment. How did Jung get around these dangers in his own explorations? And in his work with others? And with his students? Did he—get around them? I would have so many questions for Jung were he here with us.

I am grateful to Michael Monhart for affording me this opportunity to discuss this fascinating and illuminating chapter.

References

Bromberg, P. (1996). Standing in the spaces: The multiplicity of self and the psychoanalytic relationship. *Contemporary Psychoanalysis, 32,* 509–535.

Ghent, E. (1990). Masochism, submission, surrender: Masochism as a perversion of surrender. *Contemporary Psychoanalysis, 26,* 108–136.

James, W. (1917). *The varieties of religious experience.* New York, NY: Longmans, Green and Co.

Part II

Power and the social unconscious

Chapter 3

Enactment, power, or play in Jessica Benjamin's clinical theory

Ruth Imber

For more than three decades Jessica Benjamin has been a seminal force in shifting psychoanalysis from a drive-dominated theory to one focused on object relations. Her writings reflect her wide-ranging interests spanning infant development, feminism, philosophy, social criticism, and of course psychoanalytic theory. Her academic background contributes to the breadth of her knowledge. It does, however, also contribute to her writing often being challenging to read and comprehend. Benjamin makes demands on her reader. But, as I discovered by reading and re-reading some of her work, there are definite rewards for making the effort.

For a sense of her most recent thinking, I read her most recent book, *Beyond Doer and Done To* (2018). Not surprisingly, her current ideas build on those she has presented earlier. I have a need to translate some of her terminology into more familiar, and to my mind, experience near ideas. For example, the notion of 'doer and done to' seems very similar to the sorts of sado-masochistic responses familiar to most clinicians when we challenge certain patients. In response, when attacked by the patient, most of us have had the unpleasant experience of falling into the trap of defensively attacking the patient right back, often in the guise of making a 'helpful' interpretation. Identifying such an enactment is extremely useful clinically as are other of Benjamin's theoretical constructions once they are applied to our actual work.

This chapter will focus on her concept of enactments, their relation to play, and the work of undoing dissociations. Benjamin seeks to explain how we help our patients change, perhaps especially those who have been seriously, even traumatically injured by early relationships. This quest is extremely welcome and valuable as not enough of us have tried to pinpoint and prove what exactly is therapeutic in what we do. As I read her, one vehicle for change involves being receptive to the out of awareness emotional pull the patient's unconscious life scripts exert on the analyst, scripts which connect to the analyst's own unconscious wishes and needs leading to enactments that neither member of the couple notices having entered into—at least at first. Once one or the other participant does become aware of the enactment, the work of untangling, repairing, and understanding can begin, hopefully as a collaborative task. Often, if I understand correctly, this repair involves the analyst taking explicit responsibility for her part in the drama and expressing apologies especially if the patient felt hurt, attacked, misunderstood, and so on. This process, Benjamin posits, allows the patient to access warded off, dissociated experiences in a safe setting. The recognition the patient experiences when these enactments are unpacked may allow the patient to deepen her capacity for mutuality and intersubjective connection. This may be as useful an explanation as any we yet have for what happens, especially with patients who have been seriously traumatized.

Let's keep in mind that not all our patients have had deeply traumatizing childhoods. Nor do all resort to pathological dissociation to cope with unbearable affects. In fact, some patients actually have halfway decent lives before entering treatment. Furthermore, some patients require a private inner world even more than learning to share all their subjective experiences with another. As Slochower (2017) has written, not all patients can tolerate the analyst exposing her subjectivity without becoming 'derailed.' Indeed, Slochower suggests, and I agree,

> There are moments when our patients (and we) want or need to have the experience of being alone with another who stays more or less 'out of it.' To move toward what's interior and private. This desire is not always a resistance to engagement; it may represent not immaturity, but the capacity to engage with oneself.
>
> (p. 288)

So, while there is much that is useful in Benjamin's ideas, I also see some problems. For example, Benjamin apparently presumes there is a before and after when identifying enactments. However, Friedman, Smith, and others suggest the analytic enterprise may actually be composed of constant enactments, with some being more disturbing or dramatic, and therefore noticeable, than others. For instance, the work done by analyst and patient to untangle the factors contributing to their sado-masochistic exchange of 'angry bites,' to use Benjamin's metaphor, itself may be seen as an enactment. Surely the analyst wants and needs to move the work forward to do his job. And the patient may, from her subjective experience, want the analyst to own up to his contribution. Alternatively, the patient may want to please the analyst by doing the work that the analyst desires. How do we know that when these things occur the analytic couple isn't exchanging one set of unconscious needs and wishes for another? How can we be sure they aren't merely engaged in another enactment that hasn't been identified as such? I don't mean to imply that when an analyst becomes aware of making a major mistake, she should never cop to it. I *do* mean to question whether this is the engine of therapeutic change from enactment to play that Benjamin seems to be positing. Perhaps it's swapping one enactment for another. And, possibly there's no way out of this sequence. Maybe the best we can hope for is moving from those enactments that feel more malignant to those that feel more benign.

Another problem, for simplicity sake, I'll call the love enactment. I don't really believe Dr. Benjamin is advocating a love cure nor that her concept of 'the third' is a simplistic term for fusion or merger. She makes quite clear in her writing that differentiation in the dyad is as important a feature of relational analysis as finding similarity. My concern is the way in which her 'thirdness' may be *misunderstood* to denote a goal for analysis where loving feelings do away with anger between patient and analyst. To repeat I doubt this is what she intends, but nips and bites don't, to my mind, fully capture the level of rage and hatred that may be uncovered if the analyst is willing to make room for such feelings. So, being too quick to apologize or repair the rupture on the analyst's part may be read as an attempt to short circuit a full experience of the negative. I fear that her emphasis on the analyst's admission of failures, especially if made too swiftly in the name of recognition and intersubjective mutuality, may actually and ironically lead to a defense against the patient's negative feelings, especially hatred. The irony I'm driving at is that according to Benjamin if the analyst is threatened by a patient's attack and becomes defensive and self-justifying, no good will come of it. I completely agree with this. I also agree there are times when an interpretation made during such a clinical moment may serve as a subtle attack on the patient. Even if not intended by the analyst, it may function as a way to get even, consciously or not, and be experienced by the patient as vengeful. So, what am I trying to say? Simply put, sometimes it is fine, and even essential, to allow a patient to hate us without rushing to soothe or undo the supposed injury.

For that matter we analysts must recognize our own sources of anger and hate in the analytic situation. Gabbard (2000) gives us a long list of motivations for the analyst's hatred of the patient:

> First the analyst is dependent on the patient for his or her livelihood, second the patient often resists the analyst's effort to understand what's going on, third the patient's agenda is often different from the analyst's, next the patient, like a baby, insists that his or her own needs must come before the analyst's. In the transference the patient will falsely accuse the analyst of all the sins associated with mother and father. The patient will stir up longings in the analyst, sexual and otherwise, that can never be gratified. After developing an intense relationship with the analyst, the patient will terminate and disappear from the analyst's life. And last but not least,

Gabbard says "the patient will undoubtedly detect many of the analyst's shortcomings and wound the analyst's self-esteem by parading them in front of the analyst" (p. 418).

Another question, for me, involves the concept of play in adult analysis. I don't believe there is ever a clear demarcation between enactments and play. Rather I see them as descriptive terms which can be applied to an oscillating process throughout a treatment. I suspect Benjamin might agree. Ever since Freud first viewed the transference as a playground (1914), analysts have used the term play to describe the safe aspects of the analytic interaction. Karen Gilmore (2005), writing about *child analysis*, was treading some of the same ground as Dr. Benjamin when she noted,

> play differs from enactments in that it is, either implicitly or explicitly, 'make-believe.' Playing in the analytic setting establishes a space without real consequences where communication between the child and analyst can occur at the developmental level of the child in a state that is demarcated as meaningful and yet not real. While both action and verbalization are involved, what is optimally achieved is an intersubjective exchange in the mutual state of playing where transformation

of the child's anxieties and defenses can be accomplished by the analyst's clarifications, reciprocal engagement, and interpretive work.

(p. 215)

Gilmore goes on to state that a child who cannot play is at a great maturational disadvantage because play allows a child to master various important developmental tasks such as trying on gender roles and handling personal traumas.

Dr. Benjamin applies this distinction between play and enactment to our work with adult patients. I agree with her observation that enactments can both conceal or reveal depending on how productively they are analyzed. I further infer she seeks to move her patients from enactment proneness to an increased capacity to play in the analytic relationship when she writes,

> To be able to play, or learn to play, as Winnicott famously declared what we analysts and patients must do, is to make use of the paradoxical space of analysis. The most obvious paradox we require is the one that permits play by simultaneously engaging in a way that feels real and not-real, though very consequential: emotionally what happens between us [is] serious make-believe.
>
> (2018, p. 146)

I'm uncomfortable with equating the term play with unreal or 'make-believe' in adult analysis. As I read Gilmore, I think she is implying that in adult analysis the feelings aroused in enactments are no less real than in any life situation. I would suggest that when we love our analyst or hate him, it isn't make believe. Rather the analytic frame allows these feelings to exist in a safe state. If the analyst is ethical and competent, sex doesn't happen and blood isn't spilled. One might just as easily say that when we move beyond an enactment, it is not to a land of make believe where the patient feels 'oh this is not real' but rather to a place where the patient can more maturely view herself as straddling the past and the present. It was real but that was then and this is now. Transference is repeating but not, therefore, make believe. Nor am I sure what's gained by calling on paradox in such a case.

It seems to me one could just as easily say that adult functioning is enriched when it grows beyond a rigid, even paranoid adherence to the reality principle and expands to allow greater access to creativity and fantasy. And, I wonder if this is some of the underpinning of what Benjamin is getting at with her use of the word play. While she overtly references Winnicott in her theorizing, I detect a kind of Loewaldian belief in the value of allowing fantasy to enrich reality that underlies Benjamin's notion of play and the dialectic between what is real and unreal. Writing about the good analytic hour, Loewald (1975) says,

> The progression in such an hour is quite similar to the progression of a work of art, a poem, a musical composition, a painting, at a propitious moment or period during the artist's work. There, too, it is the momentum of an active imaginative process which, as it were, creates the next step, propelled by the directional tension of the previous steps. This directional tension is the resultant of the artist's imagination and the inherent force of his medium. A word, a sound, a color, a shape—in the case of dramatic art an action—or a sequence of these, once determined, strongly suggests the next step to be taken. In the mutual interaction of the good analytic hour, patient and analyst— each in his own way and on his own mental level—become both artist and medium for each other. For the analyst as artist his medium is the patient in his psychic life; for the patient as artist the analyst becomes his medium. But as living human media they have their own creative capabilities, so that they are both creators themselves. In this complex interaction, patient and analyst—at least during some short but crucial periods—may together create that imaginary life which can have a lasting influence on the patient's subsequent actual life history.
>
> (p. 297)

I'll end with a reminder to us all. Evidence is required to back up our assumptions about what it is we do that helps our patients. Too often we assert when we should hypothesize. We need to demonstrate our efficacy through more research. One concept for which there is now therapeutic validation across various modalities is the therapeutic alliance. The quality of the relationship between therapist and patient is profoundly central to positive outcome regardless of the theoretical position of the practitioner. Luborsky in the 1970s as well as others subsequently have demonstrated that the strength of the therapeutic alliance is an essential predictor of success in various psychotherapies *including psychopharmacology*. I see Benjamin's sensitive attention to repairing ruptures in the relationship as being squarely in the tradition of establishing and maintaining the therapeutic alliance.

Peter Fonagy's description of mentalization-based treatment, which increases the capacity to 'recognize' the mental states of other people and our own, reminds me a lot of what Benjamin is talking about. Alison and Fonagy (2016) identify three components of the therapist's attitude they believe are essential if treatment is to be beneficial: humility, patience, and acceptance of different perspectives. They come to the conclusion that all effective therapies result in an increase in 'epistemic trust.' Like a securely attached baby, patients who develop epistemic trust in their therapist come to believe that they can reliably learn from him or her. This is a very important aspect of what I believe Benjamin's 'moral thirdness' contributes to her patients' growth. I hope I have that right and would welcome her thoughts on this as well as on my other comments.

References

Alison, E., & Fonagy, P. (2016). When is truth relevant? *The Psychoanalytic Quarterly*, *85*, 275–303.

Benjamin, J. (2018). *Beyond doer and done to: Recognition theory, intersubjectivity and the third*. London and New York, NY: Routledge.

Freud, S. (1914). Remembering, repeating and working through. *Standard Edition*, *12*, 145–156.

Gabbard, G. O. (2000). Hatred and its rewards: A discussion. *Psychoanalytic Inquiry*, *20*, 409–420.

Gilmore, K. (2005). Play in the psychoanalytic setting: Ego capacity, ego state and vehicle for intersubjective exchange. *Psychoanalytic Study of the Child*, *60*, 213–238.

Loewald, H. (1975). Psychoanalysis as an art and the fantasy character of the psychoanalytic situation. *Journal of the American Psychoanalytic Association*, *23*, 277–299.

Slochower, J. (2017). Going too far: Relational heroine and relational excess. *Psychoanalytic Dialogues*, *27*, 282–299.

Chapter 4

The power principle

The shame of the father or the emperor's new clothes

David Braucher

Introduction

I began researching for this chapter in hopes of getting a better grasp of a phenomenon I had been observing among the fathers in my practice. Although these fathers shared feminist ideals regarding their wives and women in general, they seemed to hold themselves singularly responsible for providing for their families in a manner more commensurate with a traditional masculine role and a belief in a patriarchal system of the past.

Presenting as rather modest, dependable guys, these patients appeared to demonstrate an unconscious presence of paternal omnipotence. This was most evident when they found themselves falling short of the ideal; they became mired in shame, self-recriminations, and suicidal ideation. The more they suffered, the more they seemed to champion a monolithic imago of fatherhood, as if it was not the cause of their shame but the undergirding of any hope of redemption. I wondered where this bastion of omnipotence originated and how it was maintained despite the absence of grandiosity in how they typically presented vis-à-vis the external world.

Although I began researching for this chapter to help understand my experiences with male patients, it is important to note that females who assume the traditional father role in their families seem to exhibit similar tendencies. The 'father' is a designation that represents a role independent of the gender of the one fulfilling the role. Perhaps this explains why my two-year-old daughter often refers to any person who may act like a father as 'Daddy,' whether that person is a man, woman, or older child. The designation represents the role she expects them to fulfill.

The self as father: Born through relationship

Thinking about the self-experience of fatherhood, I was reminded of my good-byes with my own father at the end of my visits when I was a young adult. I would walk him to his car, and he would stand there at the driver's side door—he stood in the middle of 14th street and just looked at me on the sidewalk. He smiled his crooked smile with tears rolling down his cheeks, surrendering to the moment, to his feelings. As a young adult, I was baffled. If it hadn't been a Sunday night with streets empty, and if I hadn't been feeling the warm glow of a martini or two, I would have felt terribly embarrassed. Instead, I just observed his moment. A moment that my presence seemed to instigate, and that as a young adult I was too oblivious to understand.

I had forgotten about those encounters with my Dad until my patient Steve told me about driving his car, alone, with his infant daughter. She is in her car seat in the back. As he checks on her through the rearview mirror, she gazes out the side window at the scene passing by, unaware of being seen. Steve is suddenly overwhelmed by a swell of emotion. The road up ahead blurs through his tears; he starts to sob. He pulls over to the side of the road and crumbles. She brings him to his knees.

What was Steve reacting to? Was it her vulnerability—swaddled in the trust conveyed by her lack of concern about where she was going and how she was getting there, the perils of the road outside, a parallel universe outside her purview? Or was it her obliviousness to his gaze that pulled him to realize the assignment implicit in her assumption that she was and would be cared for? Her seemingly infinite fragility was at once humbling and empowering, as if it were in an inverse ratio; the more vulnerable she was, the more he knew he would do anything to protect her. Maybe he was experiencing the birth of a self, a subjectivity coming alive. As Levinas teaches us, experiencing ourselves as a "subject is from the outset the responsible self *hostage* to the other" (Marcus, 2007, p. 517). Davis (1996) explains, "[t] he exposure to the Other is the bedrock of ... selfhood; it is the condition of subjectivity, not an aspect of it" (p. 80). This understanding of the self is fundamental to interpersonal psychoanalysis as conceived by Sullivan.

The interpersonal field

In Sullivan's (1955) understanding of the interpersonal field, he argues that we get to know ourselves through our interactions with others.

Experiencing ourselves within the field, our sense of self continuously shifts in response to emotionally charged events with others. The interpersonal field impacts our experiences and conduct with one another. It is a constant, ubiquitous, and unavoidable aspect of human existence. It pervades every moment of everyone's life. No one exists outside a field; therefore our sense of who we are is dependent on the interpersonal field in which we find ourselves. Elsewhere, I argue that the loss of an intimate relationship entails not only the loss of the other's continued presence in our lives, but also the loss of the concomitant self-experience attending that relationship (Braucher, 2018b).

Levenson (1982) extends Sullivan's concept by insisting that it is impossible to be constantly aware of how our conduct is transformed by the field. The field is a dynamic process whose impact is continuously in flux. Our experience of it is always changing so that we can never completely understand its effect. Not only is our sense of self dependent on the field, but we can only ever just begin to appreciate its impact and therefore how our self is being continually transformed by it. The field that my daughter creates often leaves me feeling like a cherry picker, as she treats me as a tool with which she can escape her diminutive size.

Rovelli's quantum perspective

The physicist Rovelli (2017), through his understanding of quantum theory, develops a similar concept of the self, stating that "[t]he nature of a man is not his internal structure but the network of personal, familial, and social interactions within which he exists. It is these that 'make' us" (p. 135). Rovelli compares the self to a wave or a mountain, which he explains are not single entities. They are simply ways that we have of slicing up the world to understand it and to speak of it more easily. "What is a wave, which moves on water without carrying with it any drop of water? A wave is not an object, in the sense that it is not made of matter that travels with it" (Rovelli, 2017, pp. 135–136). Similarly, the atoms that make up our bodies flow in and away from us. Like waves, our bodies and sense of self are comprised of a flux of events: "we are processes [which are] for a brief time … monotonous" (Rovelli, 2017, p. 136). We are systems that continually interact with the external world. We don't have a self that enters into relationships, but rather we have relationships that comprise a self.

The self-experience of fathers is created by the dynamic field they are engaged in with their children, their co-parent, and society. It is not that fathers experience themselves as good enough fathers, but we are *allowed* to feel like good enough fathers by others' reactions to us. We can call ourselves father. We can think of ourselves as being fathers, and yet, isn't this a conceit? Isn't it a common fallacy to think of ourselves as having static properties of self? After all, our self-experience is always in flux, constantly subjected to the interpersonal field, to what we are experiencing ourselves doing and how we are being treated. The father gets to know himself as powerful because he is perceived as powerful by his child and co-parent. His power is bestowed upon him by his child. The power of the father exists only in the eyes of his child. Paradoxically, the father's experience of himself as powerful renders him dependent on the child, vulnerable to receiving his own power. This is what I will refer to as the 'power principle.'

One morning, before we adopted our daughter, I awakened in a state of discombobulated anxiety. The images from my dream had dissipated quickly but left me with a powerful emotional residue of heightened nervousness. I immediately thought "how can I ever become a father?" "I can't handle my *own* life—I have to tell my husband that we have to forget about adopting a child." Thankfully, the following morning, I awoke with a dream image of a young towheaded girl looking up at me with eyes that told me that I was her father. *And I felt like I was her father.* It occurred to me at that moment that a significant aspect of the self-experience of being a father, how we experience ourselves, is dependent upon the relational reality of being experienced as a father by the other. I wondered if I could find support for this idea among theorists who have attempted to explain the role of the father. I was surprised to discover that, implicit in Kohut's concept of the *idealizing selfobject*, the fathering one's self-experience is constitutive of the child's perception of him, despite Kohut not having been an interpersonal theorist.

Kohut's idealizing selfobject

In Kohut's (1971) self psychology, we learn that the maternal function is the *mirroring selfobject* and that the paternal function is the *idealizing selfobject*, which sounds—at first blush—rather symmetrical. What is somewhat obscured in this formulation is the discrepancy between subject and object in these two modes of relating; there is a discrepancy with regards to agency. The mother, as subject, does the mirroring; she mirrors the child, the object. She claims the child as her own and pursues her connection to this child by placing the child in the center of her universe, giving the child a self image as he or she progresses, developing abilities. On the other hand, the child, as subject, does the idealizing of the father, the object. The *idealizing selfobject* is *claimed* by the child. The father permits the child to define him. The child gives the father his power, his image of himself as a protector, and provider, his image of himself as a father. According to the power principle, the powerful father is paradoxically powerful through his passivity.

Winnicott (1960) famously argues that there is no such thing as an infant without maternal care. I am arguing that there is no such thing as a father without a child to perceive him as such. The child not only makes the man (or woman) a father, but within the field between the child and the parent, a father is created. As a tearful young expectant father recently explained,

> I don't know what I was thinking, but I just realized that our child is going to look at me to be her father, she is going to look up to me the way I look up to my own father.

What is implied in my patient's statement and in Kohut's *idealizing selfobject* germinates from what Freud (1913, 1923) referred to as the paternal principle.

The paternal principle

Starting with *Totem and Taboo* (1913) and further developed in *The Ego and the Id*, Freud (1923) maintained that an "individual's first and most important identification [is] his identification with the father in his own personal prehistory" (p. 31). According to Freud's paternal principle, this identification is to a phylogenetic, internalized father: we are born with it. It is an unconscious presence that predates any relationship with an actual father and exists separate from him. It is a psychic formation that anticipates the actual father's third-party role as a separator of mother and child.

According to Freud (1913, 1923), we are born anticipating the presence of the father. This implies that the mother-infant dyad has an implied third from the beginning. Similarly, the 'baby watchers,' Fivaz-Depeursinge and Corboz-Warnery (1999), found that the basic unit of intimate relationships also contains a third, leading them to coin the term *the primary triangle*. Herzog (1980) developed the concept of "father hunger" to describe the child's longing for the absent third in his study of fatherless boys.

Studying boys with night terrors, Herzog (1980) discovered that the boys developed a fear of their own aggression as they desperately wished for their absent fathers—that despite never knowing their father, they had a desperate longing for him. I chronicled this type of aggression and longing as it became manifest in a fatherless preadolescent boys' therapy group (Braucher, 1998).

The Babadook and father hunger

The movie *The Babadook* (Ceyton and Kent, 2014) powerfully portrays the dynamics of father hunger and the paternal principle. In it, a single mother struggles to raise her spirited son after his father is killed in a car accident while driving the mother to the hospital for the delivery. As the mother attempts to maintain a consistent maternal loving presence, she is overwhelmed by her son's disruptive behavior. We observe the collapse of the family structure in an unsettling scene, as the six-year-old boy lies in his mother's bed spooning her from behind, with his leg over hers, like a lover.

As the mother fails to set limits regarding her son's misadventures, the small family becomes increasingly isolated; they become social outcasts. One night, at bedtime, the mother reads the son a book entitled *The Babadook*—a book that has mysteriously appeared on his bedroom shelf. The Babadook is a phantasmagorical creature that has many incarnations, although it often takes the form of a black silhouetted figure with a top hat. The opening line of the book reads, "If it is in a word or a look, you can't get rid of the Babadook." The child becomes increasingly fixated on the Babadook; he sees it in his night terrors as a menacing presence, like the embodiment of his father hunger.

For the mother, the Babadook takes the form of her late husband. As she attempts to deny its presence, she effectively makes the Babadook more powerful, and eventually succumbs to being possessed by it. Possessed, the mother now reacts to her son's disobedience with an unbridled rage. The boy, terrified, insists, "You are not my mother." At the climax of the film, in a moment of possession, the mother almost stabs her son. But coming to her senses, she turns her rage onto the Babadook. By acknowledging the Babadook in this way, she subdues it and protects the life of her son. After a lapse of time, we see that the family life has stabilized. The boy is calmer and more obedient. The Babadook is kept in the basement in the care of the mother. She has contained him within the home and apparently within herself.

Although initially the Babadook possesses the mother with a rage akin to an archetypal tyrannical father figure, the mother learns to modulate her newly found anger: She is able to use it to set limits and restore order to the home. Like many single mothers, she embodies the paternal principle, simultaneously straddling the tasks of both parents for her child.

According to Freud (1913, 1923), the paternal principle is inherent in our psyche. In the movie, this is portrayed by the inexplicable presence of the book in the boy's room, and the mother's inability to get rid of it. As an inborn component of our psyche, we must assume that the outward manifestation of the paternal principle is, first and foremost, a transferential illusion; he exists in the eyes of the child, the beholder. From a relational perspective, we might say that as the boy is haunted by his *father hunger*—the Babadook—as a manifestation of the paternal principle, his resulting behavior interpersonally incites his mother to embody the paternal principle and set limits on her son.

Lacan's le nom-du-père

Lacan's (2006) concept of the le nom-du-père—the name of the father—is a *master signifier*: it represents an absolute law—one that cannot be truly understood and cannot be destroyed. Much like the Babadook, it has an absolute and sublime presence as well as symbolic significance. And like Freud's paternal principle, le nom-du-père, does not have to do with the actions of an actual father, but rather with the disembodied functions associated with his role with which the child is unconsciously identified.

In elaborating on the paternal principle, Lacan conceives of le nom-du-père as the means by which the child is introduced to the symbolic realm—the world of meaning. Lacan points out two important aspects of le nom-du-père: the limit setting and naming functions. The law of the father—the father's 'non'—inhibits the child's Oedipal desire for exclusive possession of the mother. The naming function entails the father giving the child a surname—his or her 'nom'—thus identifying the child within the social sphere, providing an identity in the world apart from the mother. In this sense, this paternal function gives birth to the individual, just as naming an object throws it in relief from the raw unmediated sensory experience of the reality that surrounds it and imbues the object with signification. It allows for differentiation from the mothering one and provides the basis for self-awareness by opening a space between symbol, symbolized, and the observing self (Ogden, 1992; Braucher, 2018a).

The paternal principle and the transference illusion

The role of the paternal principle in providing self-awareness is addressed by Eizirik (2015) and Aisenstein (2015), who claim that it must be activated or reactivated in order for psychoanalysis to function. This is true regardless of whether a father had been present in the patient's earlier life. Baranger and Baranger (2008) argue that regardless of how our theoretical orientation conceives of the analytic relationship, there is always a certain asymmetry between patient and analyst, and therefore whether it is addressed or not, the paternal principle is present. After all, the analyst is the guardian of the setting; the analyst sets the frame.

It occurs to me that although the paternal principle is present regarding the frame, it may also be partly responsible for the initial positive transference that allows a patient to seek treatment. If patients don't believe that the analyst has the ability to help them and keep them safe in the process, why would they ever approach treatment in the first place? In this regard, the paternal principle functions regardless of whether the analyst is called on to assume a maternal or paternal role in the treatment.

When I was a beginning therapist working at a clinic in the Bronx, I was always in a state of anxiety on my way to work on Monday mornings. *What am I doing? I am not a therapist.* Having spent the weekend not being a therapist, I didn't know how a sense of identity, the self-experience of being a therapist would manifest so that I could do my job. But soon after the first session of the day began, I would once again regain my self-experience as a therapist. My patients, through their expectations, through their interactions with me, made the paternal principle manifest within the interpersonal field. It was a necessary aspect of my nascent self-experience as a therapist. They had a belief that I could help them, and as long as I didn't disprove this belief, I just might be able to do so. This type of transference is similar to how Freud (1900) describes his father and the principle of the Gschnas.

The Gschnas

Discussing a dream about his own father in the *Interpretation of Dreams*, Freud (1900) compares fathers to the principle of the Gschnas. In Viennese culture, the Gschnas "consists of creating an object of rare and valuable reputation out of trifles, and preferably out of comical and worthless material" (Freud, 1900, p. 216). As Weineck (2014) describes in her book *The Tragedy of Fatherhood*, the Gschnas is "a comical hodgepodge, an imitation object of great repute that on closer inspection consists of worthless trifles" (p. 169). According to this description, the father is not only primarily a transferential illusion, but he might only exist within the illusion of the transference. A closer look reveals that he is an illusion made of refuse. It is perhaps because of this that Weininger (1980), as cited by Weineck (2014), concluded that "[f]atherhood is a miserable delusion" (p. 17). It is a delusion born out of a child's illusion that collapses once the child is disillusioned. In other words, *the child giveth, and the child taketh away.*

The impotent father

The Oedipus complex and the father: The other side

If the father's power exists only in the eyes of the child, how does the father maintain a positive self-experience of himself as a father when the child acts as his rival during the Oedipus complex? For Freud (1910), the resolution of the Oedipus complex is the main achievement of the psychosexual stages of development. According to Freud (1910), the child accepts being denied the fantasy of possessing the mother, of replacing the father. This is described by many as the basis for the child's perception of the father as tyrannical rival and victor, but for the father—himself—this must feel like anything but a victory, unless he is the type of man capable of relishing the pyrrhic victory of besting the child in his care. In her reading of Lacan (1977), Weineck (2014) concludes that "[t]he father may be the figure of omnipotence to his young children, but never to himself, and least of all, perhaps, in gazing at his child" (p. 166).

Moreover, it seems to me that to assume that the child ever really wanted to possess his or her mother in the same way this child's father does would be what Ferenczi (1949) referred to as "a confusion of tongues." If Ferenczi is right, and a child's desires or fantasies express a different type of sexuality than an adult's sexuality, the notion of the Oedipal complex becomes muddied, along with the accomplishment heralded as its resolution. To this point, Searles (1972) asserts that Freud ignored the day-to-day reality of parenting in which the child possesses the mother in a pervasive way. The child cries at night and the mother comes running. The child has the stay-at-home mother to him- or herself all day. The male child does not get to take the father's place in sexual relations, but what does this actually mean to a little boy? He gets something much more important. He is her constant preoccupation. He is the recipient of her physical, emotional, and psychic affection. The father gets what is left over after mother's nightly visits to the nursery.

Along these lines, a mother recently told me a joke shared among her friends.

> If you have to throw either your husband or your child off a cliff who would you throw? Before having children, the wives say, "my child," but after they have children, they don't hesitate to *toss their husbands off the cliff.*

Laius complex

With that in mind, it is not surprising that Ross (1982) found that many men feel left out of the mother-child dyad. This led him to speculate that while the child has an Oedipal complex, the father has a reciprocal Laius complex. According to Sophocles' version of the myth, it is Laius who sets the tragedy in motion. After being informed by the soothsayer that his son would eventually kill him and take his wife as his own, Laius sends his son to die from exposure in order to save himself and his relationship with his wife. Ironically, to avoid the prophesied tragedy, Laius inadvertently facilitates it. Having been sent away to die, Oedipus does not know the true identity of his biological parents, so he unknowingly kills his father and marries his mother. According to Ross (1982), as the boy has a rivalry with his father, the father has a reciprocal rivalry with his son, as he experiences his infant son displacing him from his previous privileged position vis-à-vis his wife, the mother.

Ross (1982) uses Laius to express his belief that filicidal inclinations are universal among fathers. Although everyone can fantasize about killing their child, I don't know if this qualifies as an inclination to do so. But more importantly, Civitarese (unpublished manuscript) might encourage us to go a step further. In his paper on "Rage and Shame," he explains how shame is often at the root of rage. If being a father gives rise to rage, it might be more productive to look for what is causing the shame.

According to Ross (1994), not only must the father cope with being excluded from the mother-infant dyad, but his own sense of phallic power is, in actuality, a defense against womb envy. In a recasting of the Oedipal complex, Ross (1994) surmises that the boy eventually identifies with the father, but with a feeling of loss and resignation. In Ross's view, the power residing in the phallus is a defense against the powerlessness felt in the face of the more significant maternal power. I would add that this sense of powerlessness is exacerbated by shame at failing to embody the imago of the powerful patriarchal father.

Lacan's square root of minus one

The powerful imago of the patriarchal father is often symbolized by the phallus, as a master signifier. Lacan (2006) explains that a master signifier is the square root of minus 1, "$S = \sqrt{-1}$ " (p. 694). In mathematics, the square root of minus one is known as an imaginary number. It is necessary to make certain calculations, but—in the end—it is a fiction, not a real number. In fact, it is an impossible number. According to Sauvayre (personal communication, October 17, 2017), implicitly comparing the erect phallus to an imaginary number, Lacan appears to place the erect phallus squarely in the realm of the imaginary register. In fact, when we talk of phallocentrism, we think of things like tall skyscrapers or rockets, not slinky, droopy appendages. The powerful phallus, as we imagine it, is erect, a state that often requires some form of stimulation provided by the other. Moreover, the achievement of this prominent state cannot be sustained for more than four hours at a time without requiring medical attention. On its own, the phallus most often remains diminutive and flaccid, and perhaps more comfortably hidden beneath a fig leaf.

Womb envy

Lacan of course was not the first to argue against overvaluation of the phallus. As early as 1927, Jones postulated that males envy the mother's creative power. But of all the analysts, Karen Horney (1924, 1932), laid the greatest stress on how a son's awe of his mother contributes to a sense of inadequacy as he desires to be strong like her. Horney attributed man's degradation of woman to his intense longing to control the mother's power.

Fromm (1943) also described this dynamic. He asserts that men are envious and fearful of women for their capacity to reproduce naturally. "[D]espite all his economic and sadistic and phallic superiority, man could not fail to discover that the [women] possess a unique power over mankind. She [can] produce children *who always* [*cling*] *to her*, who [love] her without stint" (Zilboorg, 1944, p. 288, italics added).

The fading patriarchy

Fromm's (1943) understanding of man's awe of women's reproductive power is probably the best rationale for the patriarchy. According to this logic, the patriarchy functions to accommodate the disparity between men and women in the domestic sphere, and to ensure the dominance of men. As the logic goes, if women are deemed property to be controlled by their husbands, then men can have some control of women's power over mankind. It also allows men the comfort of knowing that their wives are bearing *their* children. The patriarchy specifies a societal structure for fatherhood, rendering the father responsible for the children of his wife.

Historically, "[t]he father's position was defined by social and political relations that designate his body as having been there [during conception]" (Weineck, 2014, p. 82). Before the advent of DNA paternity tests, biological paternity was assumed by the father being married to the mother. In this sense, although men were the head of the household, fatherhood was not the principle of the household but a product of it. It was, and still is, marriage that confers paternity. The children of a man's wife are understood to be his own, and marriage is—of course—regulated by the state.

Therefore, fatherhood still requires institutions to give it legitimacy. According to New York law, birth fathers may be invited to participate in the adoption process, but it is not required. If fathers aren't married to the mother, they don't even need to be notified that they ever had a child. Furthermore, despite the seemingly scientific nature of DNA paternity tests, the impact of the results is adjudicated by a court of law. In these ways, fatherhood continues to be determined by the state, and each time political structures change, the fate of fatherhood comes into question.

The ancients

Although many political thinkers have played with the definition of father-hood, Plato's is most surprising (Weineck, 2014). Plato proposed abolishing fatherhood altogether to create a just state without private property. He surmised it would be better if children were raised communally. In his rebuttal, Aristotle argued that we take better care of our own possessions than we do of what we own in common.

As Aristotle attempts to describe the subjective experience of fatherhood, he employs a number of metaphorical comparisons, the sum of which add up to a paradoxical quagmire that may be the best description of fatherhood I have ever read. According to Weineck (2014), Aristotle considers

> What kind of relationship can you have with somebody who is simultaneously a separate body and an extension of your own? Someone who is somewhat like your best friend and somewhat like your teeth? Someone you ought to rule in the same way that your mind rules your soul, and your soul rules your body, but who, unlike your slave or your tooth, will take your place?
>
> (p. 106)

Although one may argue that motherhood suffers from a similar quagmire, motherhood comes with an unbroken biological chain of custody wherein the mother gets to experience the child growing within, exiting her body, and then using her body for nourishment. There is a primary biological relationship between mother and infant that is simply not afforded fathers. Fathers may or may not remember the act that led to conception. Fatherhood has always suffered from uncertain paternity and perhaps more importantly from paternal uncertainty due to the power principle. This is implied in Freud's concept of Vatersehnsucht.

Vatersehnsucht

In Freud's myth of the primal horde, the brothers succeed in killing the tyrannical father, only to resurrect him as a totem—a symbol of the law—a law that ensured that no one brother took the place of the father (Freud, 1913). As the brothers all agreed to relinquish the position of the father, they could live in a democracy in harmony with each other. "Paternal power, according to this formulation depends on the empty space the actual father left behind, creating what Freud calls Vatersehnsucht, the guilty longing for the father that can cathect to any powerful male figure actual or imagined" (Weineck, 2014, p. 174).

When paternal power is predominantly a psychic effect in the mind of the child that can attach itself to any role model, the actual father's paternal subjectivity is one of uncertainty. It is the nature of fatherhood, of being a role model, to be replaced by another. This leads to what Weineck (2014) refers to as the "father series," the personal set of role models an individual adopts to replace the father and subsequent father figures.

Castrating paternity

Weineck (2014) argues that "[h]aving to embody the function of the symbolic father, the real father's experience is one of mute surrender, making the voice falter in a mouth full of mush" (p. 167). In elaborating on Federn's (1919) notion of a *fatherless society*, she concludes, "There is no paternal subject: Federn's patriarchy knows only sons (and occasionally daughters), and the fathers have no inner life of their own—they are, in fact, coterminous with the state itself and equally faceless" (p. 180). The dilemma for men is that they can no longer embody the position of being the patriarchal father but are still expected to fulfill the role.

In modern society "[t]he great anxiety besetting ... men is not the fear of the castrating father but the fear of becoming the father, paternity, in turn emerges as nothing but a different form of castration" (Weineck, 2014, p. 170). Just this year, I had two expectant fathers in my practice voice their concern that once their child was born, their lives would be over; they would no longer be able to pursue their creative pursuits and realize their dreams. As society becomes more interested in innovation rather than tradition, the power goes to the rebels, the young, the innovators. As the son in Turgenev's novel *Fathers and Sons* takes his intellectually trendy, learned friend as his new role model, his elderly father laments, "He has cast us off; he has forsaken us, ... forsaken us ... Alone, alone!" (Turgenev, 1901, p. 112).

The relational turn

Freeman (2008) writes, "psychoanalytic theory recreates the fundamental paradoxes of patriarchy by giving a central place to the father as a symbolic figure of authority while eclipsing men's relationships with their infants under the shadow of the omnipresent nurturing mother" (p. 114). According to Winnicott (1960), the father's role is to sustain the mother-infant dyad by providing the structure with which the dyad is protected and maintained within the greater society. Winnicott's formulation seems to depend on the patriarchy remaining in place. Without the patriarchy sustaining men's hierarchical place in society, fatherhood becomes the rickety scaffolding that skirts the edges of a firm family foundation of the mother-infant dyad, with the mother as the true phallus, the real seat of power. The father is in a supporting role: the servant by the door awaiting orders.

If men are not artificially sustained by a patriarchal system, then how do we accommodate their lower status in the family? Making women equal in and out of the home leaves the role of men wanting—currently sperm can be grown in a petri dish. Somehow a father has to be strong and able to stand alone *and* lose his wife to his child while being excluded from the mother-infant dyad. How does a social animal cope with being an outsider in one's own home and yet remain related without the support of the company of men and the power bestowed by the patriarchy?

Looking at this from an intersubjective perspective of mutual recognition, we must recognize how the failing patriarchy is affecting men. For the millennia of the patriarchy, men were the doers and women were their possession, the done to. In a crumbling patriarchy, men's source of power is dissolving. Benjamin (1988) argues that masculinity entails disowning and projecting dependency needs onto women giving them an excess of dependency. But it seems to me that there is also a reciprocal dynamic occurring in which independence is being projected onto men, and men suffer from an excess of perceived independence, an expectation of independence, all the while shamefully suffering an unacknowledged dependency on their children for a sense of power. While feminism urges us toward female equality, all things are not equal. We want equality for women, but we still want men to be men. As Edward Tronick explained for a recent *New York Times* article, we still teach boys to just "man up," whereas girls are encouraged to talk about their feelings (Reiner, 2017).

Strindberg's (1887) play, *The Father*, depicts this tendency in stark relief. The wife threatens to send the couple's only daughter away to school against the father's wishes. She is taken aback by his reaction and exclaims, "What! You are crying, man!" (p. 42). The father responds,

Yes, I am crying although I am a man. But has not a man … senses, thoughts, passions? Is he not … hurt by the same weapons. … If you prick us do we not bleed? … And if you poison us, do we not die? Why shouldn't a man complain, a soldier weep? Because it is unmanly? Why is it unmanly?

(p 42)

Unable to acknowledge his manhood in light of this emotional entreaty, his wife responds, "Weep then, my child, as if you were with your mother once more" (p. 42). Later, the wife concludes, "Now you have fulfilled your function as an unfortunately necessary father and breadwinner, you are not needed any longer and you must go" (p. 44).

I think it is important to keep in mind that just because the patriarchy is bad for women, it is not necessarily good for men. As evoked by Strindberg (1887) and argued by Gilligan and Snider (2017), both genders are victims of the gender binary's maintenance of the patriarchy. Men, as well as women, are in the position of being done to. Women must relinquish their agency and men are constrained to forego their need for relatedness in order to conform to societal expectations. Gilligan and Snider (2017) wisely place the patriarchy apart from either of the sexes and understand all in society to be subjected to it. Their answer is to resist conforming to the gender binary.

In my experience, this resistance is already underway among the 'woke' fathers in my practice. However, as these men perceive women as equal in every way, it doesn't seem to affect their need to embody the model of their own internalized patriarchal fathers. Ross (1982) explains that "[f]atherhood awakens a productive identification with [a man's] own father, who now replaces his mother as the nurturing and creative figure to whom he can liken himself" (p. 11). The new father creates an image of himself as a paternal caretaker by identifying with the caretaking qualities of his own father. The father is not only subjected to how he is perceived as a father by his child and partner, but also the positive ways he remembers his own father. There is a personal historical dimension that persists beyond any father's personal attitude toward the patriarchy or feminism. Like the Gschnas, the father's image of himself as a father is "cobbled together of bits and pieces, some useful, some obsolete, a bricolage of fear and desire a repetition of memories … of ancient [myths] and fading [ideals]" (Weineck, 2014, p. 174). Despite being forward thinking feminist supporters, fathers rely on the past to construct an image of themselves as fathers. As Faulkner (1919) famously asserted, "The past is not dead! Actually, it's not even past" (p. 85).

Enter Trump

So, what happens when fathers are stuck between a crumbling patriarchy, the loss of their paternal authority, and their tendency to identify with the fantasy of the powerful fathers of their childhood? Shame, opioid addiction, an increase in middle-aged white male suicide, and Donald Trump.

Trump's supporters stand by him—not despite his erratic behavior, but *because* of it. They perceive him as strong. He is not politically correct. He says what he feels like saying as if he doesn't care what other people think. He can grab any woman at will. He is shameless. This is actually a fitting description of the father of Freud's myth of the primal horde. Apparently, for Trump supporters, the primal horde brothers' experiment in democracy has gone awry; having foregone usurping the role of the primal father, they have lost their power entirely. Trump represents the return of the despotic primal father, the tyrant.

Ross (1983) argues that to be able to cope with all the feelings engendered by fatherhood takes a self-assured man, one "who can look back upon his life and at the future with a feeling of value and purposefulness" (p. 313). When employment, the means of feeling valuable and purposeful in a capitalist society, is not available, a man might desperately turn to the hope promised by a charlatan, someone who guarantees that he alone can fix it, that he alone can take care of it. You only have to believe him. In this, Trump is actively playing on the power principle, the father born out of another's perception, the father who derives his power by being perceived as powerful. Maybe this is why he continues to hold rallies after becoming president: he needs to re-experience his power within the interpersonal field; he needs the refueling.

Paternal omnipotence

As discussed above, fatherhood is an embodied illusion born of the earliest days of a child's projection and a new father's submission to that projection. Whereas women experience their motherhood as both physically and socially conferred, men must rely solely on being socially engaged into experiencing fatherhood. Whereas maternal power comes from a woman's experience of herself creating a child within her womb, paternal power is bestowed by the child and is subject to being taken away by the child, as the father is replaced by newer, cooler role models.

Patriarchy has functioned to keep men engaged with their children by conferring paternity and offering the support of the company of men, but—as such—it has always been a support that is subject to change according to political will. As the awareness of women's subjugation has evolved, many men are no longer comfortable viewing women as less than equal. Yet gender equality brings hidden problems. One might say that patriarchy was a solution to a problem and—without it—the problem has returned.

According to Ross, "fatherhood does away with the vestiges of outworn illusions of parental omnipotence, ... exposing one's parents as simply frail individuals" (Ross, 1983, p. 312). A sentence later, he adds, "a new father searches for actual memories and fantasies about himself and his father—and mother—from which to recreate a representation of an *all powerful 'good' father*" (Ross, 1983, p. 312 italics added). According to Ross, with the awareness of our own father's lack of omnipotence, a new illusion is quickly reborn to take its place—the all-powerful father. Being a father entails believing that we can be what we know we can never be. It is like the emperor's new clothes; we not only admire them although we don't actually see them, but we need to see them so badly we find ourselves disbelieving our own eyes.

The fathers: The paternal bastion

For many of the fathers in my practice, this illusion seems to take a form similar to what Baranger and Baranger (2008) refer to as a bastion: an unconscious, unresolved circumscribed belief in one's own omnipotence. However, it is different than their typical bastion in that the paternal bastion is not solely intrapsychic. The omnipotence of the power principle occurs within the interpersonal field. It is a self-experience of power bestowed on the father by the child and, at times, by the mother. When this power is no longer interpersonally bestowed, the blow to the father's identity results in shame. As Lynd (1958) discovered in her sociological study, shame is the result of finding ourselves falling short of how we think of ourselves, how we self-identify.

Hank

Hank first came to treatment at the insistence of his mother following the death of his father, an abusive alcoholic who provided for the family financially, but who was more likely to make Hank feel endangered than safe. He was a gruff man who demanded obedience but allowed no access to his interiority. What Hank knows of him is what he surreptitiously observed. He came to know of his father as emotional only after he caught a glimpse of him through a crack in the door to the family room, sobbing with a scotch, while listening to John Philip Sousa's "The Stars and Stripes Forever." He saw his father slam the arm of his chair and point up to the ceiling. This eccentric, emotional tyrant took his secrets to the grave with him along with Hank's hope of understanding the father of his childhood.

As a young father, Hank forestalled his budding career as a musician in order to avoid being on the road for long periods of time. He wanted to be a part of his son's daily life. He so longed to feel and to be a part of his son's early life that he found a lactation specialist to help him rig a tube to a container of formula so he could experience himself feeding his son as his son sucked on his finger. The experience of himself as a father in the early days rivaled the joy of being appreciated for his musical talent. His son's excitement at his arrival home from work rivaled the applause of a cheering crowd, filling him with a sense of value and purpose.

In these early years, it was easy for Hank to feed his own father hunger by being an available father to his son and, two years later, to his daughter as well. He woke them for school and made breakfast in order to have time with them. Later, during his son's early adolescence, Hank would wake him an hour earlier so they would have time to play the guitar together. His son looked up to him as an accomplished musician and wanted to be like him. Hank became a soccer coach for both his son and daughter's teams, relishing being witness to their developing abilities.

Now, as Hank's son progresses into late adolescence, he has put down the guitar. He would rather hang out in the neighborhood with his soccer friends than play guitar or go camping with his father. No longer experiencing himself through the lens of the power principle, which was so apparent in his son's early years, Hank imagines he did something wrong. His son no longer looks up to him as a role model for their shared interests.

Bereft of his close relationship with his son and the loss of his obvious importance to him, Hank shared a recent fantasy that if his son unwittingly got his girlfriend pregnant, Hank would raise the child himself, a chance at a *do-over*. Blaming himself for their increasingly distant relationship, Hank imagines that, somehow, he could have done things differently. In his omnipotent fantasy, he could raise a child who would never replace him with new role models. When Hank shared this fantasy with his wife, she quickly pointed out that the son's girlfriend's family would probably claim the child; after all, she would be having the child. As the father of Strindberg's play laments, "A man has no children, it is only a woman who has children, and therefore the future is hers when we die childless" (Strindberg, 1887, p. 55).

As Hank's son prepares for college, the growing family's expenses begin to strain the budget his languishing music career provides and Hank feels like even more of a failure as a father. His financial contributions pale in comparison to his father's corporate salary. Although, realistically, Hank is aware that he made career sacrifices in order to be present for his children in a way his father never was, his appreciation of this fact doesn't compensate him for his shortcomings as a provider at present. Prompted by his unconscious omnipotent fantasy, Hank believes he should be able to do it all, but at the very least he should be able to provide for his children the way his father did, and that also means doing it alone: he is the sole breadwinner.

Hank is impressed with his wife's success as a community organizer. She is a member on a number of community boards with close connections to local politicians. But neither Hank nor his wife have ever considered that she should find a paying job. Hank explains that he and his wife were raised with stay-at-home mothers and with fathers who provided financially for the families. This is his image of a father, a remnant of his childhood father imago and an image that is fortified by his wife's own father imago. It is Hank's shame that he has failed to embody the image of a successful provider.

Fortified by the intimacy of our six-year analysis, Hank has become more familiar with the impact of his unconscious omnipotence and has grown to better tolerate his vulnerability without shame. Mourning the losses he suffered regarding his own father of childhood, and now his son, has allowed him to reach a level of acceptance that has rendered his omnipotence less despotic. Though the unconscious omnipotence remains,

Hank's ability to identify its manifestations has greatly reduced the sting of the shame and sense of failure they once engendered. As he identified with the emotional sustenance he received from me in the transference, he grew to better appreciate how the emotional commitment he made to his children provided them with lasting psychic nutrients he never received from his own father. As he is often visibly moved by swells of pride in how his children turned out, I encourage him to enjoy these crucial moments of parental narcissism. Though relatively sobering, he knows that what he *has* accomplished is a viable expression of a *relatively potent* self.

John

John is in a similar position. When he was worried about his job security and his ability to maintain the family in the manner to which they were accustomed, he felt he must suffer in silence. He could not convince his wife that they could not afford to rent a summer home in Spain for her and the children, while he remained in the city to work. He felt it was his job to provide for the family—to share his fears with his wife was to fail at his role and to burden her with his shame. The fact that his job was in jeopardy—in part due to his taking time off to care for a newborn so that his wife could go to school to study for a year—was immaterial. It was his responsibility to provide for her and the children. Failing to do so brought shame that overcame him until he developed the suicidal depression that landed him in treatment.

Russ

Russ also has a capable wife with a law degree who opted to stay at home and care for their two boys. She works a non-paying job for the local school board, which Russ appreciates as a difficult job doing good for the community. He, too, would never suggest that his wife get a paying job to help support the family as the boys enter college. Russ's father was a benign patriarch, and Russ is the heir apparent, impregnated with a sense of omnipotence. When this unspoken, unacknowledged omnipotence was challenged by a heart condition that required open heart surgery and months away from work, Russ developed intrusive suicidal thoughts. On his return to work, balking under the pressure of his own self-expectations, he would find himself standing on the train platform thinking, "just jump!"

As with Hank, the work with John and Russ involved learning about and mourning the loss of the sense of self that was motivated by unconscious omnipotence. Appreciating their own fathers as good enough, but flawed, helped weaken the grip with which their unconscious omnipotence routinely crushed their self-esteem. As the erosion of shame abated, they were fortified to more openly share their concerns with their wives, enlisting them as true partners in meeting the challenges of providing for the family. The once shameful proof of their failure as fathers to be suffered alone in isolation became the bedrock of partnership.

Karl

Karl prided himself on being a provider for his family, his wife, his two children. Unbeknownst to his wife who turned a blind eye toward the family finances, Karl ran into financial trouble and was in considerable debt. Soon after he took his life by jumping out the window of their apartment, his wife came to me for treatment to deal with her grief and to try to understand how this happened so completely outside of her awareness. Although much of what happened remains shrouded in mystery, all seem to agree that Karl determined that he was worth more dead than alive. A generous life insurance policy that paid out even in cases of suicide has more than covered the debt and has left his family able to maintain their comfortable private school lifestyle and to pay for college for the two children. Unfortunately for his wife and children, he did not value the importance to them of having a living father.

Conclusion

In each of these men, just a sampling from my practice, there is a monolithic image of the father to which they feel compelled to realize and—at times—necessarily fail to embody. This is their shame, their deep shame. Since none of these fathers present as grandiose, rather seem to be fairly solid, humble guys, I can only imagine that their paternal omnipotence exists sequestered in their unconscious as it does not impact the rest of their personalities. But unlike an interpsychic bastion, their unconscious is activated by the interpersonal field of the power principle, in which paternal omnipotence is relationally initialized by the women and children in their lives. Maybe the 'father hunger' that Herzog discovered in children exists in all of us to a certain extent, awaiting the next available target to which to attach. As long as that target does not reject our idealization, it takes hold. Although this target could be a woman as easily as a man, I wonder if men are more commonly socialized to embody this type of projection. Masculinity's drive for autonomy over relationship seems to prime men to empathically engage with this projected image. When this image is no longer interpersonally maintained by his children, his wife, and society, the result is the shame of the father.

Epilogue

I'm two and a half years into my experience of fatherhood and my previous life is a distant memory—vague and colorless. Not that it was dull before, but now, my life is so completely altered, it holds little in common with the past. Having our daughter has reoriented our lives like a powerful magnet being dropped among a handful of metal shavings. These lines from "Anecdote of the Jar" by Wallace Stevens (1919) perhaps expresses it better:

> I placed a jar in Tennessee,
> And round it was, upon a hill.
> It made the slovenly wilderness
> Surround that hill.
>
> The wilderness rose up to it,
> And sprawled around, no longer wild.
> The jar was round upon the ground
> And tall and of a port in air.
>
> It took dominion everywhere.

Whatever else the poem brings to mind, it is evident that the presence of the jar has transformed 'the field' of its surroundings and "took dominion." Its mere presence changes the nature around it. And our daughter, like the jar, placed in our home, changed the nature of our relationships to ourselves.

My husband and I have always had strong personalities, and although we don't hesitate to say, "No," to our daughter, her very presence has a gravitational pull that orients us, reduces us to satellites in orbit around her. When she was an infant, although she was the easiest of babies, I found myself preoccupied with all the dangers that might befall in her life. She seemed so perfect and pure, I feared the challenges she might face that might tarnish her happiness, deform her as only life experiences can. I worried about everything from mean girls to randy boys, from creepy men to the existential effects of global warming. As Judy Garland says in the new biopic *Judy* (Livingston & Goold, 2019), having a child is "like wearing your heart on the outside of your body."

Now, though, as she's a toddler, I take joy in witnessing her ever-evolving abilities; I also long for the days when I could put her down and find her in the exact same position when I returned. Now walking, and climbing, and falling, her fragility is my liege. And when I have to say, "No," although I know it is for her safety, it feels like anything but power. The tears streaming down her little cheeks reach a soft spot deep inside me, and I fear I am the one doing the damage.

I have never put myself into debt, apart from mortgages and student loans, and yet, having a daughter feels like I have incurred the debt of my lifetime: I owe my whole life, and hopefully, a long life, to making sure that she is safe, secure, and cared for. To adopt her was the one decision that would determine all the others that follow.

Since we decided that my husband would forego his career to be a stay-at-home parent, I have taken on the responsibility of providing for the family. Whereas I never struggled with providing for myself, I also always had the freedom to know that I could adapt to whatever changes in fortune came my way. Now, I know that any changes in fortune would have an immediate and formative impact on her, leading to a telescoping of consequences that will extend beyond my lifetime—with any luck. It is only in a funhouse mirror that this could be experienced as a position of power. Although I am grateful to be privileged enough to be able to provide, the need to provide is experienced as an imperative, inexorable. This is the paradox of the power principle; it is a power that can only be truly experienced as accountability, of knowing one is engaging in an impossible task that can only result in relative failure. Yet one doesn't hesitate, can't hesitate, to keep at it. (Note: to the extent this experience is the same for mothers, they, too, can be subject to the power principle.)

Acknowledgments

I would like to express my sincere gratitude to Pascal Sauvayre, Warren Wilner, Jill Gentile, and the editors-in-chief of *Contemporary Psychoanalysis* for their valuable contributions.

References

Aisenstein, M. (2015). The question of the father in 2015. *Psychoanalytic Quarterly, 84*, 351–362.

Baranger, M., & Baranger, W. (2008). The analytic situation as a dynamic field. *International Journal of Psychoanalysis, 89*, 795–826.

Benjamin, J. (1988). *The bonds of love: Psychoanalysis, feminism and the problem of domination*. New York, NY: Pantheon Books.

Braucher, D. (1998). Darth Vader v. Superman: Aggression and intimacy in two preadolescent boys' groups. *Journal of Child and Adolescent Group Therapy, 8*, 115–134.

Braucher, D. (2018a). A therapeutic dyad in search of a third. In R. C. Curtis (Ed.), *Psychoanalytic Case Studies from an Interpersonal-Relational Perspective* (pp. 209–212). London, UK: Routledge.

Braucher, D. (2018b). Passion of past-shunned: The use of fantasy to recreate past loving and sexual self-experiences in the present. In B. Willock, R. C. Curtis, & L. C. Bohm (Eds.), *Psychoanalytic perspectives on passion* (pp. 195–202). London, UK: Routledge.

Ceyton, K. (Producer), & Kent, J. (Director). (2014). *The Babadook* [Motion Picture]. Australia: IFC Midnight.

Davis, C. (1996). *Levinas: An introduction*. Cambridge, MA: Polity Press.

Eizirik, C. L. (2015). The father, the father function, the father principle: Some contemporary psychoanalytic developments. *Psychoanalytic Quarterly, 84*, 335–350.

Faulkner, W. (1919). *Requiem for a nun*. London, UK: Chattq & Windus.

Federn, P. (1919). *Zur psychologie der revolution. Die vaterlose gesellschaft*. Leipzig and Vienna: Anzengruber Verlag.

Ferenczi, S. (1949). Confusion of the tongues between the adults and the child— (The Language of Tenderness and of Passion). *International Journal of Psycho-Analysis, 30*, 225–230.

Fivaz-Depeursinge, A., & Corboz-Warnery, A. (1999). *The primary triangle: A developmental systems view of mothers, fathers and infants*. New York, NY: Basic Books.

Freeman, T. (2008). Psychoanalytic concepts of fatherhood: Patriarchal paradoxes and the presence of the absent authority. *Studies in Gender and Sexuality, 9*(2), 113–139.

Freud, S. (1900). The interpretation of dreams. *The Standard Edition of the Complete Psychological Works of Sigmund Freud, Volume IV (1900): The Interpretation of Dreams (First Part)*, ix–627.

Freud, S. (1910). A special type of choice of object made by men (Contributions to the psychology of love I). *The Standard Edition of the Complete Psychological*

*Works of Sigmund Freud, Volume XI (*1910*): Five Lectures on Psycho-Analysis, Leonardo da Vinci and Other Works*, 163–176.

Freud, S. (1913). Totem and taboo. *The Standard Edition of the Complete Psychological Works of Sigmund Freud, Volume XIII (1913–1914): Totem and Taboo and Other Works*, vii–162.

Freud, S. (1923). The ego and id. *The Standard Edition of the Complete Psychological Works of Sigmund Freud, Volume XIX (1923–1925): The Ego and the Id and Other Works*, 1–66.

Fromm, E. (1943). Sex and character. *Psychiatry, 6*, 21–31.

Gilligan, C., & Snider, N. (2017). The loss of pleasure, or why we are still talking about Oedipus. *Contemporary Psychoanalysis, 53*(2), 173–195.

Herzog, J. (1980). Sleep disturbance and father hunger in 18- to 28-month-old boys—The Erlkönig Syndrome. *Psychoanalytic Study of the Child, 35*, 219–233.

Horney, K. (1924). On the genesis of the castration complex in women. *International Journal of Psychoanalysis, 5*, 50–65.

Horney, K. (1932). The dread of woman. *International Journal of Psychoanalysis, 13*, 348–366.

Jones, E. (1927). The early development of female sexuality. In *Papers on psychoanalysis* (pp. 438–451). Boston, MA: Beacon Press, 1961.

Kohut, H. (1971). *The analysis of the self*. New York, NY: International Universities Press.

Lacan, J. (1977). The function and field of speech and language in psychoanalysis. In *Ecrits: A Selection*. (A. Sheridan, Trans.). New York: W. W. Norton.

Lacan, J. (2006). *Ecrits*. (B. Fink, Trans.). New York, NY: Norton.

Levenson, E. A. (1982). Follow the fox—An inquiry into the vicissitudes of psychoanalytic supervision. *Contemporary Psychoanalysis, 18*, 1–15.

Livingston, D. (Producer), & Goold, R. (Director). (2019). *Judy* [Motion Picture]. United Kingdom: Pathé & BBC Films.

Lynd, H. M. (1958). *On shame and the search for identity*. Oxford, UK: Harcourt, Brace.

Marcus, P. (2007). "You are, Therefore I am": Emmanuel Levinas and psychoanalysis. *Psychoanalytic Review, 94*(4), 515–527.

Ogden, T. (1992). *The matrix of the mind*. London: Maresfield Karnac.

Reiner, A. (2017, June 15). Talking to boys the way we talk to girls. *The New York Times*. Retrieved from https://www.nytimes.com.

Ross, J. M. (1982). Oedipus revisited—Laius and the "Laius Complex". *Psychoanalytic Study of the Child, 37*, 169–200.

Ross, J. M. (1983). Father to the child: Psychoanalytic reflections. *Psychoanalytic Review, 70*(3), 301–320.

Ross, J. M. (1994). *What men want: Mothers, fathers and manhood*. Cambridge, MA/London, UK: Harvard University Press.

Rovelli, C. (2017). *Reality is not what it seems: The journey to quantum gravity.* [Kindle Edition]. Retrieved from http://www.amazon.com.

Searles, H. F. (1972). Unconscious processes in relation to the environmental crisis. *Psychoanalytic Review, 59*(3), 361–374.

Stevens, W. (1919). Anecdote of the jar. *Poetry, 15*(1), 8.

Strindberg, A. (1887). The father. (E. Oland and W. Oland, Trans.) [Kindle Edition]. Retrieved from http://www.amazon.com.

Sullivan, H. S. (1955). *The interpersonal theory of psychiatry*. London, UK: Tavistock Publications Limited.

Turgenev, I. (1901). *Fathers and sons*. (K. Casey, Trans.) [Kindle Edition] Retrieved from http://www.amazon.com.

Weineck, S. (2014). *The tragedy of fatherhood: King Laius and the politics of paternity in the west*. New York, NY: Bloomsbury.

Weininger, O. (1980). *Geschlecht und charakter: Eine principielle untersuchung*. Munich: Matthes & Seitz.

Winnicott, D. W. (1960). The theory of the parent-infant relationship. *International Journal of Psycho-Analysis, 41*, 585–595.

Zilboorg, G. (1944). Masculine and feminine. *Psychiatry, 7*, 257–296.

Chapter 5

Enacting identity

Normative unconscious processes in clinic and culture

Lynne Layton

In this chapter, I will talk about the psychological effects of power structures and socially constructed hierarchies that contain within them judgments about human worth, about what counts as human. My focus is on how these social hierarchies affect the ways in which our identities are formed and interpersonally performed. Most of the chapter focuses on identity formation in the context of hierarchies of gender, race, class, and sexuality, but I will also speak briefly, at the end, about some broader socio-historic trends that affect subject formation and the way we experience and enact our identities. My hope is that we can think together about what it might mean to talk about a social unconscious or, in terms that highlight process instead of substance, what it might mean to talk about unconscious processes that are deeply inflected by social norms. In particular, I'd like us to consider how these processes play out in clinical interactions and enactments.

I begin with a cautionary tale. A few years ago, I was asked to comment on a paper written by Lawrence Kubie (Layton, 2011; reported in Layton, 2020), a prominent analyst during the 1950s and into the early 1970s when he died. Just after he died, *The Psychoanalytic Quarterly* published one of his papers, titled "The Drive to Become Both Sexes" (Kubie, 2011; orig. 1974). In 2011, *The Psychoanalytic Quarterly* decided to reprint the paper with commentaries by Ken Corbett (Corbett, 2011) and myself. Kubie had begun giving this paper from the 1950s on but for some reason had never felt comfortable publishing it until the early 1970s. Kubie's theory was that some people, and many artists, have a neurotic drive to be both sexes; this drive, he felt, was crippling and highly resistant to analysis. He described several vignettes with patients suffering from this illness. In one example, he spoke of a male patient who, he said, was rather passive and not at all competitive. He then likened this man to an adolescent girl (p. 387), implying that adolescent girls are passive and not competitive, and that real men are supposed to be non-passive and competitive. Kubie's interpretations reflected his adherence to the strictly binary, white middle-class gender norms of the 1950s. These norms were articulated in many discourses, for example, in prominent sociologist Talcott Parsons' family theory (Parsons, 1949). Parsons lauded as natural and most desirable a social system that divided men and women along the axes of instrumental, breadwinner roles and expressive, caretaking roles. Kubie's work suggests how such mainstream gender ideology can find its way into clinical theory and practice. For example, in a lengthy vignette, Kubie described a female patient of his who

> had a flair for writing, a fine dramatic gift, and great warmth in her attitudes toward children. In the course of her treatment she went through successive phases—working on the stage, writing, and teaching in nursery schools. … She did each extraordinarily well; yet each also carried its multiple and conflicting meanings.
>
> (p. 421)

Kubie went on to say that

> For many months secret, lifelong fantasies of going on the stage had been completely absent from her material. Then as she approached the end of her analysis, she suddenly fulfilled a prophecy that I had made silently to myself by turning once again toward a stage career. This was buttressed by excellent rationalizations, including high praise from her dramatic coaches and her successes in certain competitions. *Her battle became … whether to have children or to have a stage career; or to put it another way, to be one sex or the other or both.*
>
> (p. 421, my emphasis)

Here is a dream from the end of this patient's analysis with Kubie. In the dream, the patient

> was auditioning for the role of Blanche Du Bois in *A Streetcar Named Desire*. … In the dream, having auditioned successfully for the role

of this unhappy psychotic prostitute, she wandered away. Then she stooped to pick up a half-dollar. But it was not a round half-dollar piece; it was one half of a round dollar, a half-moon. She picked this up, looked at it, and dissolved in tears.

(p. 422)

Kubie concluded, "In the course of time, with this warning in mind, I returned her to analysis with a woman, with whom she carried her therapy through to successful completion" (p. 422).

On reading this, I, too, just about dissolved in tears. From the vantage point of having experienced the second-wave feminist movement that was, at that very moment, in the process of deconstructing the gender norms Kubie was unknowingly enforcing, I could recognize that this woman and the previously mentioned male patient were being asked by their analyst to be half a human. As I said, Kubie's diagnosis of these patients was that they suffered from the drive to be both sexes, a diagnosis that, as you can see, is not just descriptive, but prescriptive. In his interpretations, Kubie, we could say, was performing a strict gender binary. As Judith Butler (1990) has taught us, repeated utterances of the diagnosis, and the repeated interpretations dictated by the diagnosis, are precisely what end up legitimizing the gender binary that makes half-people out of whole people. To put it psychoanalytically, the diagnosis and interpretations legitimize the splitting processes that one would have had to undergo in order to occupy a position culturally recognized as properly male or properly female. Looking again at Kubie's cases, we can say that to perform the gender binary 'correctly,' a proper male is expected to split off passive strivings, dependency longings. A proper female should want to have children and give up any notion of a career. To want a career is to want to be male, evidence of the drive to become both sexes. The interpretations Kubie derives from the diagnosis are thus not the neutral or universally true statements he believes they are; rather, they enact and thus enforce particular sexist and heterosexist social norms of the day. As I discuss in more detail below, I see such enactments as evidence of what I call normative unconscious processes.

I found Kubie's paper infuriating but also heart-wrenching—heart-wrenching because I knew that Kubie had gone over and over this paper for 20 years before publishing it. This gave me the feeling that Kubie might himself have suffered from this so-called drive to be both sexes and might have also attempted to exorcise from himself longings that are human longings: to be caretaking and taken care of, to be autonomous and have your autonomy recognized as legitimate by another, to be dependent and passive and not be humiliated for it.

It is easy to feel horror when listening to work like this, and all too easy to feel we are beyond enacting such egregious sexism in our clinical work. But I begin with Kubie because I do not think it is fruitful to consider what he did as a 'mistake.' Rather, I begin there because his theorizing and his work, undoubtedly characteristic of his era, caution us to think deeply about the way that mental health experts can unconsciously enforce and unwittingly legitimize only those performances of identity deemed proper by the culture and subcultures in which we live. In my experience, it is in fact not as uncommon as we might hope, even today, to hear case presentations in which human attributes like assertion and dependence are gendered.

One way that people have thought about what is operating in examples such as Kubie's is to imagine the existence of a social unconscious that structures our identities and permeates the consulting room. Erich Fromm (1941, 1962, 1970), an early interpersonalist and an early member of the Frankfurt School, perhaps the first group to attempt a synthesis of Marx and Freud, proposed two mechanisms by which the social world becomes part of the individual's unconscious. First, he thought that the social unconscious consisted of everything we repress in order not to be aware of social contradictions, socially produced suffering, the failure of authority, and feelings of social malaise and dissatisfaction (Fromm, 1962, p. 131). And the reason he thought we repress such awareness and feelings was fear—not fear of castration or annihilation, but fear of social isolation and ostracism (1941, p. 126), a fear of losing social approval and a sense of belonging, of losing love. For most people, Fromm wrote, identity is rooted in conformity with social clichés; to be aware of the truth is to risk loss of identity.

Gary Walls (2006) gives an example of a political awareness barrier breaking down and then quickly reasserting itself because of fear of social isolation and punishment. As he and his daughter walk toward their coach airplane seats, they pass through first class and his daughter asks if their seats are there. His first thought is to tell the truth as to who travels in first class and what first class is about. Multiple and contradictory feelings begin to consume him, but fear of getting kicked off the airplane and fantasies of being interrogated by Homeland Security make him just say, no, honey, our seats are further back, with no explanation but lots of feelings of shame.

Second, Fromm (1941), like Wilhelm Reich (1933/1945) and others, also developed the concept of social character, that is, the typical character structure and typical defenses of a particular culture. Psychosocial attempts to account for fascism in Germany led Fromm and other members of the Frankfurt School to investigate an authoritarian personality marked by a split between submissive behavior toward authority figures and tyrannical behavior toward intimate others (see, Fromm, 1984, and Adorno et al., 1950). In the late 1970s and early 1980s, Christopher Lasch (1979) and Joel Kovel (1980), following in this social character tradition, drew on Kohut (1971, 1977) and Kernberg (1975) to write about narcissistic character and a culture of narcissism. But until recently, few theorists, either within clinical or applied psychoanalysis, have written about how unconscious processes shaped by our experience in the social world are present in clinical work. I want to mention a few mediating concepts from the academic and clinical worlds that have facilitated my thinking about the way that socially inflected unconscious processes emerge in the clinic: the concept of the social construction of identities within particular power hierarchies, the concept of identities as performative, and the concept of enactment.

The social construction of identities

Some years ago, a dear friend of mine had fraternal twins, a boy and a girl. I went to the hospital the day after they were born, and, to me, they looked identical. During the visit, their father picked up the boy and said, "Is this a boy, or what?" Thinking "or what," I realized on the spot how impossible it would ever be to separate nature from nurture in understanding the development of something like gender identity. I began to be aware of how differently people talked to and held girl babies versus boy babies; I read Stephen Seligman's (1999) work on how unconscious parental projections into infants begin from day one—even in utero—as anyone can attest who's been to a baby shower where the gender of the child is known. What the projections are will of course differ depending on one's personal history, one's historical moment, and one's class, race, sexual, religious, and other identifications, but this only renders more complex and relational the process of social constructions of identity.

Here is another example drawn from everyday life (reported in Layton, 2020). On another visit with friends, we invited guests learned that their eight-year-old daughter Emily had been making movies with her nine-year-old male friend. We visitors quickly discerned that the proud parents wanted us to watch the movies, so watch them we did. Although I was prepared to be bored, I found *Lovestruck I, II*, and *III* to be an astounding trilogy, in which Emily and Joe had enacted a rather sophisticated presentation of class, race, sex, and gender conflicts. The theme of these three movies was the social barriers to the love between an upper-class white girl and a lower-class white boy. At first, the young lady, draped in an adult's fur boa, told her single dad, played by her father, that she was repelled by this "boy," whom they both call an "amateur" (which seemed to be their word for lower class). The boy earns her love by being good to his mom and the best student in the class; as they work on their projects together and she comes to see how very considerate and ambitious he is, the cold and distant emotional shield she has erected against whatever it is she considers to be associated with the poor begins to erode.

In all three films, money worries feature prominently. *Lovestruck III* concerns the financial difficulties they face in their married life. Attention is diverted from this problem when Emily is kidnapped by a lower-class black thief who shows all of the attributes of poverty against which Emily had erected her upper-class defenses in the first place—he's unkempt, loud, boorish, takes rather than earns money, and is a sexual predator. A happy ending resolves the tensions but also masks the fact that the film's social conflicts are unresolvable—and that they are psychic conflicts as well.

Emily, under the influence of whatever goes on and has gone on in her intergenerational family, in her school, and in her peer group, is struggling to find her way into a classed and raced position. Her fantasy suggests that this position is created and maintained by splitting off certain ways of expressing feeling and certain kinds of desire, by disallowing certain kinds of activity, and by dehumanizing whole classes of people. Her conflict about her raced class position, which may involve such psychic phenomena as guilt over privilege or a longing to be able to enact some of the forbidden behaviors associated with the black lower class male of her fantasy, or anger and confusion at her family's concern with money, is expressed in part in her desire for the poor boy. The conflict is managed in fantasy by the way she gives him the attributes that make him safe for marriage (i.e., the attributes that make him a good bourgeois, including his whiteness).

The failure of her attempts at management surface in the appearance of the black kidnapper, who grabs sex and money without guilt. Emily and Joe are clearly working out problems that beset their culture and their families and that have become part of their psychic legacy. Their story reveals how genders become classed and raced; the intersectional social construction of identity apparent in *Lovestruck* also shows the way that the emotions and psychological structures that we work with every day in therapy—dependency, assertion, vulnerability, emotion—become gendered, raced, classed, and sexed in the process of identity formation; and how identities lived in conformity with various social inequalities play out in relation. Subjectivity and relationality, in short, are psychosocially constructed.

Identities as performative

In the early 1990s, Judith Butler (1990) revolutionized ways of thinking about identity by positing a performative theory of gender identity. This theory suggests that femininity, for example, is not an internal substance that expresses itself in the world; rather, femininity consists of repeated performances of culturally established gender norms, like ways of speaking, walking, talking, dressing, that, because so often repeated, come to *feel* like something internal to female subjects. Butler's theory led to some wild individualist interpretations, in which various gender performances were understood as something one could don or discard according to whim. Butler (1993) was then at pains to insist that some performances of gender are culturally encouraged and some are utterly tabooed—think of the Kubie examples, in which interpretations perform the assumption that there is something innate that is clearly masculine or clearly feminine, and that the two are mutually exclusive. When we introduce into the picture the operation of power structures, we find that the two sides of binaries like masculine/feminine, straight/gay, white/black, are not equally but rather differentially valued. The first in the pair is often endowed with all the characteristics idealized by dominant culture and thus valued more highly. The 'other' in the pair is not merely different, A versus B, but rather deficient, lacking something, holding all the characteristics of lesser value, A versus minus A. For example, what is male is rational, female emotional. What is white is enterprising, and what is black is lazy. Cultural hierarchies figure difference in terms of distinctions between superior and inferior.

Although in Butler's early social constructionist work, any notion of internal psychic structure was denied or downplayed (Layton, 1998, Ch. 8), her later work (e.g., 1995) is more properly psychosocial. Here, she examined the psychic effects of binaries and recognized that what is performed is conditioned by what has been tabooed. In other words, identifications are unstable and often bear the psychic trace of prior disidentifications and of parents' own unconscious conflicts transmitted to the child. Butler grounds her theory in Freud's discussion of mourning and melancholia (Freud, 1917), and the idea that the ego is built up of loved and lost object cathexes, some of which are culturally allowed to be mourned and some of which are not. Performances of heterosexuality, she argues, are conditioned by a *prior* cultural taboo on homosexual desire: the negative Oedipal phase of same-sex desire is culturally disallowed and the loss is not allowed to be mourned and grieved. These losses and taboos bring into being the culturally sanctioned Oedipal demand, which heterosexualizes by dichotomizing identification and desire: one is to identify with the same-sex parent and desire the opposite-sex parent.

I have interpreted Butler's ideas about identity performance and constraint through interpersonal and Kleinian theories. For example, Donna Bassin (1996) presented a vignette about a woman who had become passive and incurious in her life, mentioning as formative an event in which the patient, who loved being in her mother's closet and smelling and touching her clothes, was one day discovered by her mother 'in the act' and humiliated and smacked. I understand such moments as precisely the kind that contribute to producing a heterosexual identity that rests on a taboo against homoerotic desire—in this case tied up with a taboo on curiosity (see Layton, 2000). As Butler (1995) contends, same-sex desire does not disappear but rather haunts performances of heterosexual identity, making heterosexuality a fragile structure.

Enactment and the effects of the social

'Enactment' is a clinical concept that has proven crucial to bringing into relation the psychic and the social. Many clinical schools believe that traumatic experience that cannot yet be symbolized is instead enacted. Corollary to the belief that therapeutic encounters are marked by unconscious processes circulating between patient and therapist, one definition of enactment refers to unconscious collusions within the dyad that re-enact (rather than analyze) earlier traumatic experience. Indeed, Gerson (1996) reformulated resistance in terms of such mutual collusions.

In the late 20th and early 21st century, psychoanalytic clinical practitioners, particularly those within the relational psychoanalytic and the group analytic traditions, began writing about the ways that social inequalities are re-created in and sometimes sustained by unconscious enactments in the clinic (Altman, 2000, Layton, 2002; Hopper, 2003; Leary, 2000; Straker, 2006). Various terms have been introduced to account for such phenomena: group analyst Earl Hopper (2003) describes a 'social unconscious' defined as "the unconscious constraints of social systems on individuals and their internal worlds, and, at the same time, the effects that unconscious fantasies, actions, thoughts and feelings have on social systems" (p. 126). Hopper looks for enactments of a social unconscious in group process, for example, anxiety stemming from hospital layoffs emerges in the group as conflict between doctors and nurses or between old group members and a new member. In the context of treating black freedom fighters in apartheid South Africa, white South African analyst Gill Straker (2006) speaks of an 'anti-analytic third,' which she describes as "a mindlessness generated by a particular set of circumstances that implicates our social histories as well as our personal ones" (pp. 729–730). "When present," she writes, "it produces impasses that predispose patient and therapist to see each other in socially stereotyped, mutually hurtful ways" (p. 740). Neil Altman (2000) gives a striking example in describing the way he, a white Jewish male analyst, and his black male client engaged in an enactment around payment, one that mobilized white unconscious racial stereotypes regarding the unreliability of blacks, as well as shameful feelings in the analyst and fantasies that his patient saw him as a greedy Jew. Altman and Straker think about both the social and the unconscious less in terms of substance than in terms of process, the repeated performance of particular practices and relationally, psychosocially constructed identities. Theories of dissociation and enactment complement Butler's performance theory by pointing to ways that socially inflected unconscious processes are enacted in the clinic, both by patient and therapist, and how those enactments can perpetuate binary identity structures and cultural hierarchies.

Normative unconscious processes

From the 1950s to the 1990s and beyond, a variety of social movements emerged, each influenced by the other, to demand recognition for culturally devalued identities: civil rights, second-wave feminism, black power, gay and lesbian liberation, Act Up, queer theory, and trans movements. Second-wave feminists, who at first had wholly rejected psychoanalysis as irredeemably sexist, began to experience in their relational lives sexism's deeply unconscious psychic effects, effects that perpetuated the self-oppression of even the most socially conscious feminists (see, for example, Dinnerstein, 1976; Chodorow, 1978; Benjamin, 1988). This led to a return of interest in psychoanalysis. Along with other relational psychoanalytic feminists in the 1980s and 1990s (Benjamin, 1988; Dimen, 1991; Goldner, 1991; Harris, 1991), I began to think about how culturally constructed gender binaries enforce processes of splitting and projection. My own contribution to this literature (Layton, 1998; Layton, 2002) was to focus on the psychological effects of assigning some human capacities to one side of the split and others to the other side; I also began to describe and theorize the kind of enactments in which identities are performed in such a way that social inequalities are not only expressed but reproduced. I wanted to understand what happens to the psyche when love and social approval are given only for certain ways of being human and not others, when they permit certain identifications and encourage disidentifications with what is socially considered undesirable. I wanted to understand what it is like to *live* the splits mandated by various binaries—to look at what becomes experienced as me and what as not-me and how the not-me gets projected onto others.

A patient of mine, whose father humiliated him by calling him female names and constantly suggesting he wasn't the right kind of male, told a story about overhearing his boss talking to his four-year-old son, who apparently was weeping uncontrollably on the phone (reported in Layton, 1998, ch. 7). After trying to cajole the boy to stop crying, my patient overheard the boss tell the boy to pull down his pants. He then asked, what do you see there? The boy must have said, "a penis." That's right, the boss said, so stop crying. How will this boy live the effects of coding vulnerability and emotionality as female/feminine; how will he live the demand to repudiate those states? How will it affect his relationships? A friend's father, who expected his sons all to become doctors, would taunt my friend if he got anything less than an A on exams. "What do you want to be, a truck driver?" he'd condescendingly say (see Layton, 2004a, pp. 47–48). Patricia Williams (1997) describes the psychic effects of hate learned in the context of love. What will it take for this boy to see a truck driver as human? How will this boy live the internal split between whatever of his attributes, emotions, and capacities get associated with doctor versus truck driver? How will these split states become enacted in interpersonal relationships both intimate and more socially distant? What boundaries will he need to draw between self and other in order to sustain whatever he calls his identity?

In earlier work (Layton, 2002), I used the term heterosexist unconscious to describe what was going on in enactments that sustained sexism and heterosexism. Stephen Hartman (2005) then used the term class unconscious to describe both how class is intergenerationally transmitted to become part of one's identity and how class struggles are enacted in the clinic. Noting an increasing number of clinical papers on unconscious enactments of unequal power relations, and beginning to write, myself, about class and racial enactments, I suggested an umbrella term, 'normative unconscious processes,' to describe enactments that reproduce traumatic experience related to subjects' social and historical positionings (Layton, 2006a). Normative unconscious processes are an effect of the workings of unequal power arrangements on identity formation and relational interactions. Identities form in relation to other identities circulating in a culture and subculture, and identities are in part made up of socio-historically specific ways of living emotions such as shame, sorrow and guilt, and psychological states such as dependency, vulnerability, and capacity for assertion. Norms and practices that derive from social hierarchies of sex(ism), class(ism), race(ism), heterosex(ism) mandate what counts as a 'proper' versus 'improper' identity. Recognition (in the form of social approval, love, conditions for social belonging) is granted, albeit often conflictually, to 'proper' performances of identity; the risk of meeting with indifference, humiliation, and shame discourages 'improper' performances and encourages subjects to split off as 'not-me' disapproved of ways of being and relating, ways that provoke anxiety or shame in significant others. Because, however, what gets split off in normative unconscious processes are human needs, capacities, and longings, these do not disappear; rather, they reappear in symptoms and in relational struggles.

Let us look at some examples, beginning with a return to Kubie. In the culture he describes, consonant with white middle-class norms of the 1950s, capacities for assertion and capacities for connection are split. Where, for example, assertive strivings become not-me but are still present because they are part of what it is to be human, you might find symptoms like those Kubie found. Kubie's female patients were depressed; they raged against their selfish husbands, they nagged because they couldn't express what they wanted directly, they grudgingly gave up desired careers to become mothers, and, in so doing, they sustained the masculine/feminine splits that had caused their suffering in the first place. Actions, feelings, and relational moves that sustain the splits are instances of normative unconscious processes. Counter-normative processes that seek to undo the splits are generally present as well—like dreams in which you weep as you pick up a half of a round half dollar. Note that late in that analysis, Kubie's patient again asserted her desire to be on the stage and gave the analyst one last chance to recognize the legitimacy of the desire. I would contend that subjectivity is, in part, marked by struggles between normative unconscious processes and counter-normative unconscious processes that contest the former's psychic hegemony.

I understand normative unconscious processes as effects of an intergenerational transmission of trauma, not the kind of trauma we generally think about when we think about intergenerational transmission—war, famine, political oppression—but trauma nonetheless because they result from the way that social inequalities are experienced on an individual level; they derive from experiences in which love and recognition are felt to be given in exchange for disidentifying with a part of oneself and a part of what it means to be human, where parts of self are at best unacknowledged, and, at worst, shamed.

Now I would like to turn to my own clinical work and explore how normative unconscious processes get enacted and how such enactments are sometimes worked through but sometimes reproduce social inequalities.

Sandy was born in the late 1970s, the first child of a white mother who grew up in poverty and a white father who rose from being blue collar to bureaucratic white collar (this case was first reported in Layton, 2014, pp. 464–465, and subsequently in Layton, 2020, Ch. 10). Father never let mother forget where she came from, and much of Sandy's specialness to father was wrapped up in his often-stated aspirations that she rise in class and status. Because she was so special, he asserted, she could do and have whatever she wanted. Intuiting this source of father's love, Sandy worked much harder academically than any of her peers, and she did indeed rise to become a professional in a high-income field. She thus secured her place as her father's favorite—which involved denigrating mother. What Sandy always knew, but couldn't really know until therapy, is that her father's capacities for love were rather damaged, and a part of her greatly resented what felt like a love contingent on performance. Her fragile sense of specialness was bolstered by her utter disdain for peers who didn't work as hard as she: "Someday they'll be cleaning my toilets," she thought when she saw them out having fun while she studied.

Sandy fell in love with a working-class man who himself had risen to be bureaucratic white collar. As her therapist, I listened over and over again to her mocking denigration of his working-class ways. I surmise that Sandy thought she was bonding with me and my, in her view, exalted class position when she was denigrating the classlessness of her boyfriend. But, of course, it was her own anxiety about not being classy enough that she feared would be revealed—and dreams did at times reveal it. I found it difficult to listen to how she talked about her boyfriend. At the point where I could no longer bear her contempt and could find a way to confront it calmly, I pointed out to her that she seemed to need to mock her boyfriend and we ought perhaps to look at why. The first time I brought this up, she practically had an anxiety attack on the couch. She had an instant moment of recognition that, in fact, much of her sense of who she was, her identity, rested on this defensive kind of class mockery, and she suddenly felt herself unraveling at the prospect of being shorn of this defense. It took much work to understand how her class grandiosity related to class disidentifications with mother and identifications with father's disdain for what, in mother, reminded him too much of his disowned class insecurities. She eventually came to understand how the class grandiosity was a defense against recognizing that father's love was contingent on her achievements—her mockery was aimed as much at hated parts of self that she had come to associate with classlessness as at her boyfriend.

Class wounds run deep. When it feels like love is contingent on performance, love itself gets tangled up in sadomasochistic enactments. Indeed, until she met this boyfriend, Sandy was entirely cynical about love. For years, she'd been cheating on her previous upper-middle-class boyfriend with a lower-class man she'd dated in high school—perhaps another way of externalizing and interpersonalizing her personal class struggle. But

Sandy was aided in her denigration of love by a fairly new subject position offered to professionalizing women, one formed at the intersection of neoliberalism and a middle-class version of feminism. This is a subject position in which dependency is denied and caretaking capacities devalued in favor of a single-minded focus on career goals—and, indeed, before analysis Sandy occupied this position without seeming conflict. In her determination to rise in class, Sandy had become the kind of non-relational maximizer of self-opportunity described in critiques of neoliberalism. She had come to hate her own vulnerability and to project it onto her boyfriend and lower classes in general. But we might guess that she fell in love with this boyfriend in part because he was comfortable with his class, with all she had come to call not-me, even though she would try to get me to laugh with her at him for wearing a gold chain or showing some other sign of belonging to the white working class.

Sandy's case suggests that, to sustain the identity position that had received love and approval, she continuously had to split off and project onto others the parts of self that had come to be labeled bad-me or not-me. Like Fromm, I would argue that the reason you do this damage to yourself is because it is too dangerous to lose the love and approval on which, in part, the stability of our developing identities depend. But identities formed in this way are also defensive and fragile, haunted by what has been split off. Sandy tried to enlist me as her classy accomplice, but, in this case, I wasn't pulled in. In the following cases, however, I indeed was complicit in sustaining the binary products of gender, race, sexual, and class splitting, re-enacting rather than analyzing what had caused psychic distress in the first place.

Enactment, co-construction, and the analyst's complicity

In this first vignette (reported in Layton, 2002, pp. 211–212), I believe that I 'performed' Butler's theory of how the heterosexist split between desire and identification comes into psychic being. A lesbian patient fell madly in love with me and detailed her erotic fantasies over the course of two or three sessions. In the third session, I picked up on a criticism she had made of her partner earlier in the session: she doesn't ever touch me in the right way. Only vaguely aware of the anxiety her fantasies had stirred up in me, I later said that here she didn't have to worry about me touching her in the wrong way, since here we would not become sexual. She felt shamed and she stopped talking about her sexual desire immediately. Over the course of the next months, she began to experiment with 'girly' things, clothes, manicures, that she had never tried before. This was a playful period, which I enjoyed immensely and so undoubtedly encouraged. It was only a year later, when she informed me that she wished she could wear sweatshirts, pants, and hiking boots every day—because, she said, that's who she is—that I began to think back to the 'femininity' period. I wondered if the comment I made that had ended the sexual fantasy had then led the patient to retreat from desire to identification, a way of connecting with which she thought I might be more comfortable. I am suggesting that because of my discomfort with my own same-sex desire, I perhaps brought about the performance of the culturally mandated split between identification and desire. Had I dealt with my own erotic feelings, I might have sustained with her the ambiguities of sexual desire; instead I sustained a straight/gay split that produced a masculine/feminine split. In so doing, I upheld the heterosexist norm. In this case that meant shaming the gay patient, precisely what the enforcement of heterosexual norms is designed to do.

In a psychotherapy session with an Asian American gay male patient who tended to stereotype Westerners and Asians rather rigidly, I found myself unconsciously supporting dominant racial and gender norms by feminizing him (reported first in Layton, 2006a, pp. 247–261, and subsequently in Layton, 2020, Ch. 11). Over time, he had described several situations in which he thought Westerners reacted differently from the way he did. In some instances, he felt superior to Westerners; in others, he felt inferior. For instance, he told me that when people were walking toward him on the street, he always stepped aside. His white Western boyfriend had pointed that out to him in a way that suggested he wasn't assertive enough. He was confused because to him this felt polite. But he wondered if he was being a doormat in this and other situations. At one point, I told him I was struggling to understand this dilemma. I said that I recognized that in part what he described had to do with norms of politeness that he preferred to what he called Western rudeness, but that I also recognized in what he was describing something akin to the position of female subordination to men that feminists have written about (e.g., Benjamin, 1988). As it turned out, the latter part of what was consciously meant to be an empathic comment seems to have re-ignited wounds that undoubtedly derive from the way Asian males are feminized in white Western culture and with the way gay males are feminized in heterosexual culture. I unwittingly humiliated him—to do, likely, with my own wounds generated by sexism and what it meant to be sitting with a man struggling with autonomous strivings; toward the end of the session he retaliated by telling me he was thinking of ending therapy, and then associating to the younger, more beautiful female therapist he had seen before he began his work with me.

In another moment of the same treatment, I colluded with him in upholding a fantasy that I, like all of the white boyfriends he chose, held the invulnerable position of whiteness. He longed for a position in which he would be immune to gender, racial, and other slights, and he associated that position with whiteness. I suppose I, too, long for a superior position in which I might be invulnerable, so I unconsciously accepted that designation. While it is certainly true that in our particular historical moment I am called and call myself white (as opposed to historical moments when Jews were considered non-white), it is also true that whiteness embodies a fantasy of invulnerability to which *no one* can lay claim. Once I realized that I was performing 'whiteness' to his inferior non-whiteness, I began to ask different questions of him than I had been asking. I tried then to deconstruct whiteness by helping him think about the vulnerable parts of himself that he hated, and how whiteness had both wounded him and become for him a fantasy guarantee that he would never again feel the pain of inferiority and humiliation. I wondered what ways of being had become barred for him in the process of becoming what he took to be a good Asian son of parents living in a dominant white culture.

I came to recognize that my own pretense to incarnating whiteness is precisely the kind of normative unconscious process that sustains racial inequality. Only much later did I realize that, for me, this pretense enacts an intergenerationally transmitted imperative, held by all four of my grandparents, to escape, via assimilation, the traumas of Eastern European pogroms, Western European associations of Eastern Jews with dirt and darkness, and American anti-Semitism (Layton, 2016). My 'wish' to occupy the position of 'invulnerability,' an unconscious collusion with the patient's wish, demonstrates that racism and class inequality do not only split the psyche of the subordinate; they also bolster the fantasmatic position of the dominant—and *both* parties want to hold to the fantasy that *someone* is invulnerable to pain and loss. The collusion acts as a mutual resistance to experiencing psychic pain, what Ruth Stein (2005) called a perverse pact. By claiming the whiteness my ancestors, as immigrants, so longed for, I, in fantasy, secure my attachment to those ancestral ghosts, keep them alive, remain loyal to them. To be recognized as white was, and to a large extent still is, to be recognized as American, to be safe and loved.

I once gave a talk in England that drew on vignettes like these, and someone in the audience said to me, "You make a lot of mistakes, don't you?" I suppose these could be considered mistakes, but I think of them more as consciousness-raising moments that offer the opportunity to rein-tegrate what had been dissociated in my attempt and my patients' attempts to be proper subjects worthy of love and social approval, a chance to toler-ate pain we hadn't heretofore been able to tolerate, and to turn what had been lived as an inferior/superior distinction from others into mere differ-ences unmarked by defensive psychic turmoil.

Social character and neoliberalism

Space does not permit more than just a few thoughts about contemporary social reality and its effects on identity formation. But I do want briefly to talk about neoliberalism and the subject positions it favors. I mentioned in discussing the Sandy vignette that a strange blend of the demands of the US workplace, individualizing and individualistic trends inherent to free market capitalism, and feminist demands for equality have led to the formation of a culturally sanctioned, if not culturally idealized subject position formerly offered only to middle-class men and now offered to middle-class women as well (Layton, 2004b, 2004c). This position is char-acterized by a valuing of achievement and self-fulfillment, and a devaluing of relational capacities. It is rooted in practices of neoliberal subjectivity that deny dependence and interdependence and that demand that the sub-ject become an entrepreneur of the self. Practices encouraging the devel-opment of entrepreneurial selves became dominant during the Reagan and Thatcher administrations, when social welfare for the vulnerable, for-merly seen as the responsibility of the state, began to be shifted onto the shoulders of private individuals. Privatization, deregulation, downsizing, outsourcing, the 2007–2008 financial crisis, and the dramatic increase in income inequality that the Occupy movements brought to public attention have caused tension between the demand to be entrepreneurial and the fear of falling, failing, of being disposable. All of this has created a great deal of anxiety about class status among all classes, including the middle and upper-middle classes we generally treat in private practice. Such anxiety, and how it is intergenerationally transmitted in prescriptions of what it means to be a proper human being, is well exemplified in an episode of the sketch comedy *Portlandia*. In this vignette, a pre-school boy, Grover, sits at a kitchen counter as his parents try to engage him in their performance of how important it is that he do well at his upcoming private pre-school interview. Holding up a flip chart that shows the trajectory that will follow if he successfully gets into the Shining Star pre-school, and noting that they have trademarked his name, the parents first point to a symbol representing an ivy league college. Then, pointing to a picture of a Ferrari, they tell him that this is the car he will drive if he gets into the pre-school. Finally, they hold up a flip chart denoting failure, and they begin to spew denigrating comments about the lower-class children with whom he will be consorting in public school, the dumb kids to whom he will be subjected to in community college, and the guns and drugs that will inevitably lead to jail. Grover looks increasingly depressed. Yet, when his parents ask him to say which chart he prefers, he readily agrees with them that the success chart is preferable.

The demand to be an entrepreneurial self is conveyed not only by parents but by other agents of the middle class as well. A former student who is now in her 30s told me that in her upper-middle-class elementary school, lessons were taught that were designed to humiliate the children into striving for upward mobility (reported in Layton, 2014, p. 470): in 5th grade, one of her teachers asked his students where their parents had gone to college. As each child responded, it became clear that the predominant answers were ivy league and elite schools. "Well," he concluded, "none of you is going to any of these schools because you don't work hard enough. You won't get your first choice." My student remembers that from that time forth she anxiously repeated to herself the mantra, "I must have my first choice, I must have my first choice." You can almost taste the invitation to a split state of grandiosity and feelings of low self-worth, and, indeed, this student suffered from depressions that had at their core a questioning of what she was doing—and for whom.

Psychoanalysts do not endorse the neoliberal agenda of subject formation. We know that when dependency and vulnerability are denied, the self becomes fragile and relations to others become sadomasochistic. And yet, psychoanalysts too can unconsciously fall in line with the neoliberal agenda, which is why I began with Kubie as a cautionary tale. A brief but very typical clinical example illustrates how neoliberalizing processes can unconsciously enter the clinic and how hard it is for a therapist to resist colluding with these processes.

A colleague presented a very familiar-sounding case in which a middle-class college student performed to perfection in one semester only to collapse into so much binging, purging, and alcohol abuse in the second semester that she could not complete any work and would find herself on the verge of expulsion (reported in Layton, 2014, p. 470). The student attempted to comply with parental and cultural demands to be an enterprising self but continued to fall sick from the attempt, rebelling in self-annihilating but powerfully signifying refusals. The therapist felt pulled to help the student complete her work, a very understandable reaction given the student's apparent panic about not getting her work done. But I think such a pull entails an unconscious collusion with the perverse pole of self-sufficient omnipotence to which so many of us, patients and therapists alike, have submitted ourselves in this neoliberal age. What I would argue is that we need to see as symptomatic not only the patient's alcohol abuse and binging, but also the demand on the patient to achieve, a demand that, in most cases is just accepted as normal. I think we need to help the patient look not only at the obviously self-destructive symptoms but also at her feelings about the demand to be an enterprising self. If we don't, we contribute to sustaining the idea that such pressures for performance are normal.

Therapists are too often trained to see the social context in which identities are constructed as irrelevant to the 'deep' work. We thus tend to cut off the kind of talk that places patients and ourselves in a psychosocial context (Layton, 2006b). When we do so, I think that we consciously and unconsciously normalize and thus performatively legitimize a conception of selfhood that is quite in line with the neoliberal version of subjectivity that radically splits the psyche from its formation in social matrices. Once the link between the psychic and the social is severed, the way is paved for an adaptationist ethic to take hold, in this case adaptation to the norms of neoliberal individualism.

I hope to have given you some idea of what I mean by normative unconscious processes and how they permeate our lives, relationships, and professional practices. My contention is that the more we are aware of the cultural waters in which we swim, aware of what we have split off, dissociated, and projected onto others in order to stabilize our own psychosocial identities, the richer our therapy work and personal lives will become.

References

Adorno, T. W., Frenkel-Brunswik, E., Levinson, D., & Sanford, N. (1950). *The authoritarian personality*. New York, NY: Harper & Row.

Altman, N. (2000). Black and white thinking: A psychoanalyst reconsiders race. *Psychoanalytic Dialogues, 10*(4), 589–605.

Bassin, D. (1996). Beyond the he and the she: Toward the reconciliation of masculinity and femininity in the postoedipal female mind. *Journal of the American Psychoanalytic Association, 44S*, 157–190.

Benjamin, J. (1988). *The bonds of love*. New York, NY: Pantheon.

Butler, J. (1990). *Gender trouble: Feminism and the subversion of identity*. New York, NY: Routledge.

Butler, J. (1993). *Bodies that matter*. New York, NY: Routledge.

Butler, J. (1995). Melancholy gender—refused identification. *Psychoanalytic Dialogues, 5*(2), 165–180.

Chodorow, N. (1978). *The reproduction of mothering*. Berkeley, CA: University of California Press.

Corbett, K. (2011). Gender regulation. *Psychoanalytic Quarterly, 80*(2), 441–460.

Dimen, M. (1991). Deconstructing difference: gender, splitting, and transitional space. *Psychoanalytic Dialogues 1*(3), 335–352.

Dinnerstein, D. (1976). *The mermaid and the minotaur*. New York, NY: Harper & Row.

Freud, S. (1917). Mourning and melancholia. In: SE 14:237–258.

Fromm, E. (1941/1969). Character and the social process. In *Escape from freedom* (pp. 304–327). New York, NY: Avon Books.

Fromm, E. (1962). *Beyond the chains of illusion*. New York, NY: Pocket Books, Inc.

Fromm, E. (1970). *The crisis of psychoanalysis*. New York, NY: Holt, Rinehart, Winston.

Fromm, E. (1984). *The working class in weimar Germany: A psychological and sociological study*. Oxford, UK: Berg Publishers.

Gerson, S. (1996). Neutrality, resistance and self-disclosure in an intersubjective psychoanalysis. *Psychoanalytic Dialogues, 6*(5), 623–645.

Goldner, V. (1991). Toward a critical relational theory of gender. *Psychoanalytic Dialogues, 1*(3), 249–272.

Harris, A. (1991). Gender as contradiction. *Psychoanalytic Dialogues, 1*(2), 197–224.

Hartman, S. (2005). Class unconscious: From dialectical materialism to relational material. *Psychoanalysis, Culture & Society, 10*(2), 121–137.

Hopper, E. (2003). *The social unconscious*. London: Jessica Kingsley.

Kernberg, O. (1975). *Borderline conditions and pathological narcissism*. New York, NY: Jason Aronson.

Kohut, H. (1971). *The analysis of the self: A Systematic Approach to the psychoanalytic treatment of narcissistic personality disorder*. New York, NY: International Universities Press.

Kohut, H. (1977). *The restoration of the self*. New York, NY: International Universities Press.

Kovel, J. (1980). Narcissism and the family. *Telos, 44*, 88–100.

Kubie, L. S. (1974; repr. 2011). The drive to become both sexes. *Psychoanalytic Quarterly, 80*(2), 369–440.

Lasch, C. (1979). *The culture of narcissism.* New York, NY: Norton.

Layton, L. (1998; repr. 2004). *Who's that Girl? Who's that Boy? Clinical practice meets postmodern gender theory.* Hillsdale, NJ: The Analytic Press.

Layton, L. (2000). The psychopolitics of bisexuality. *Studies in Gender and Sexuality, 1*(1), 41–60.

Layton, L. (2002). Cultural hierarchies, splitting, and the heterosexist unconscious. In S. Fairfield, L. Layton, & C. Stack (Eds.), *Bringing the plague: Toward a postmodern psychoanalysis* (pp. 195–223). New York, NY: Other Press.

Layton, L. (2004a). That place gives me the heebie jeebies. *International Journal of Critical Psychology: Psycho-Social Research, 10*, 36–50. Reprinted in Layton, Hollander, and Gutwill (2006). *Psychoanalysis, Class and Politics: Encounters in the Clinical Setting* (pp. 51–61), New York, NY: Routledge.

Layton, L. (2004b). Working nine to nine: the new women of prime time. *Studies in Gender and Sexuality 5*, 351–369.

Layton, L. (2004c). Relational no more: Defensive autonomy in middle-class women. In J. A. Winer, & J. W. Anderson (Eds.), *The annual of psychoanalysis, vol. 32. Psychoanalysis and women* (pp. 29–57). Hillsdale, NJ: The Analytic Press.

Layton, L. (2006a). Racial identities, racial enactments, and normative unconscious processes. *Psychoanalytic Quarterly, LXXV*(1), 237–269.

Layton, L. (2006b). Attacks on linking. The unconscious pull to dissociate individuals from their social context. In L. Layton, N. C. Hollander, & S. Gutwill (Eds.), *Psychoanalysis, class and politics: Encounters in the clinical setting* (pp. 107–117). London, New York, NY: Routledge.

Layton, L. (2011). On the irreconcilable in psychic life. The role of culture in the drive to become both sexes. Commentary on paper by Lawrence Kubie. *Psychoanalytic Quarterly, 80*(2), 461–474.

Layton, L. (2014). Grandiosity, neoliberalism and neoconservatism. *Psychoanalytic Inquiry, 34*(5):463–474.

Layton, L. (2016). Racialized enactments and normative unconscious processes: Where haunted identities meet. In J. Salberg, & S. Grand (Eds.), *Transgenerational trauma and the other* (pp. 144–164). New York, NY: Routledge.

Layton, L. (2020). *Toward a social psychoanalysis: Culture, character, and normative unconscious processes.* M. Leavy-Sperounis (Ed.). New York, NY: Routledge.

Leary, K. (2000). Racial enactments in dynamic treatment. *Psychoanalytic Dialogues, 10*, 639–653.

Parsons, T. (1949). The social structure of the family. In R. Anshen (Ed.), *The family: Its functions and destiny* (pp. 241–273). New York, NY: Harper & Row.

Reich, W. (1945; orig. 1933). *Character analysis.* New York, NY: Farrar, Straus and Giroux.

Seligman, S. (1999). Integrating Kleinian theory and intersubjective infant research: Observing projective identification. *Psychoanalytic Dialogues, 9*(2), 129–159.

Stein, R. (2005). Why perversion? "False love" and the perverse pact. *The International Journal of Psychoanalysis, 86,* 775–799.

Straker, G. (2006). The anti-analytic third. *Psychoanalytic Review, 93*(5), 729–753.

Walls, G. (2006). The normative unconscious and the political contexts of change in psychotherapy. In L. Layton, N. C. Hollander, & S. Gutwill (Eds.), *Psychoanalysis, class, and politics: Encounters in the clinical setting* (pp. 118–128). New York, NY: Routledge.

Williams, P. (1997). The ethnic scarring of American whiteness. In W. Lubiano (Ed.), *The house that race built* (pp. 253–263). New York, NY: Pantheon.

THE SEXUAL UNCONSCIOUS IN TENSION WITH
NORMATIVE UNCONSCIOUS PROCESSES:
DISCUSSION OF LAYTON

Katharina Rothe

It is with great pleasure that I have been engaging with Layton's ideas, and I am happy to and hope to bring to further discussion some of the ideas as I understand them.

I am going to raise a few questions and try to bring into dialogue Layton's conception of *normative unconscious processes* with conceptions of '*the unconscious*'—and finally address the question: *What may we lose when giving up the notion of 'the unconscious' in a Freudian sense*?

As two of the major points of Layton's paper I take the following insights:

- that we are all embedded in the social from the get-go and
- that we cannot but be entangled in the reproduction of societally dominant or normative unequal power relationships between groups of people.

Layton also demonstrated how we are inevitably entangled in the very processes we try to analyze—both in theorizing and in the consulting room.

It has been the project of critical theory of the Frankfurt School to grasp the inextricable intertwinement of nature and society in the human subject. Layton is taking up that project, when she states, for instance, "how impossible it would ever be to separate nature from nurture in understanding the development of something like gender identity"—or any identity, I want to add, as her paper speaks both *within* the logic of identities and of the inherent failure of this logic, when it comes to us being identical with our*selves*. If the *psycho*-logic of us coming into being ultimately comes down to splits of self and other, every split already presupposes or implies the fantasy of fusion that (retroactively) relates back to the earliest stages of infancy and ultimately might be captured with the fantasy of a paradisiacal state in the womb.

'The unconscious' versus 'unconscious processes'

I understand the criticism of a notion of 'the unconscious' as due to the risk of essentializing it—as if it were ahistorical—and the risk of reifying it. And there is much to say for not reifying it, so as to highlight the dynamic processes and their workings, (e.g., in a psychoanalytic session between analyst and patient) and not to turn the unconscious into a thing, which is the literal German Marxist term for reification: verdinglichung, literally 'thinging-it' (turning into a thing), when of course, by definition, the unconscious is a no-thing, to use Bion's pun.

Layton defines *normative unconscious processes* as

> an effect of the workings of unequal power arrangements on identity formation and relational interactions. Identities form in relation to other identities circulating in a culture and subculture, and identities are in part made up of socio-historically specific ways of living emotions such as shame, sorrow and guilt, and psychological states such as dependency, vulnerability, and capacity for assertion. Norms and practices that derive from social hierarchies of sex(ism), class(ism), race(ism), heterosex(ism) mandate what counts as a 'proper' versus 'improper' identity.

She uses "enactment" as a relational playing out of "traumatic experience that cannot yet be symbolized" in the encounter between people, e.g., analyst and patient.

I want to highlight the "yet" and ask if, once we symbolize traumatic experience, aren't we still always missing something? Isn't there stuff that always remains unsymbolizable?

Layton quotes Fromm as one of the early Frankfurt School members. With their concepts, such as the authoritarian personality, they wanted to bring to light how societal violence (both structural and executed violence) constitutively shapes an individual's very 'nature.'

Interestingly, Layton captures the 'later Fromm,' the one who had split with the Frankfurt School and Freudo-Marxism and who co-founded the interpersonal school.

> On the one hand, he thought that the social unconscious consisted of everything we repress in order not to be aware of social contradictions, socially produced suffering, the failure of authority, and feelings of social malaise and dissatisfaction. And the reason he thought we repress such awareness and feelings was fear—not fear of castration or annihilation, but fear of social isolation and ostracism, a fear

of losing social approval and a sense of belonging, of losing love. For most people, Fromm wrote, identity is rooted in conformity with social clichés; to be aware of the truth is to risk loss of identity.

But—I want to ask—are the two mutually exclusive? Does not the fear of losing love and recognition presuppose fears that are even more existential and corporeal and that concepts such as fear of castration and annihilation try to capture?

I am now going to take up a few examples of Layton's paper, starting with the case of Kubie (1974) and his *diagnosis* of the *drive to be both sexes*. Layton points out that this

> is not just descriptive, but prescriptive. In his interpretations, Kubie, we could say, was performing a strict gender binary. As Judith Butler has taught us, repeated utterances of the diagnosis, and the repeated interpretations dictated by the diagnosis are precisely what end up legitimizing the gender binary that makes half-people out of whole people.

At first, I found myself enjoying frowning upon and dismissing as naive and obsolete the blatant sexism in psychoanalysis of the 1950s. … But then I started following my associations and fantasies … hhmm, wouldn't it be marvelous if we could be *whole*, whole as in complete as in ful(l)filled, not so vulnerable, completely dependent and helpless upon birth, struggling for some mastery, some autonomy—in addition to wanting to be loved and recognized—just to lose all of it again at the end of our lives. Doesn't the fantasy of half people and "whole people" also speak to a desire of having it all and being it all, of wanting to be whole and not so full of holes (with an h), metaphorically speaking and no pun intended?

No matter how hard we try to analyze the social processes we are ourselves entangled in, we also imbue them with something more, this layer of fantasy—including unconscious fantasy—the kind of surplus that thinkers of 'the unconscious' have been trying to capture. What I want to get to is that we are constantly grappling with something that 'by nature' not only escapes us, but the moment we think we captured *it*, we are once more in the grip of it. And this is something I would like to demonstrate with the following examples.

Layton gives an example of a racialized enactment around payment between "a white Jewish male analyst and his black male client." This enactment, she writes,

> mobilized white unconscious racial stereotypes regarding the unreliability of blacks, as well as shameful feelings in the analyst and fantasies that his patient saw him as a greedy Jew. (Altman and Straker think about both the social and the unconscious less in terms of substance than in terms of process, the repeated performance of particular practices, and relationally, psychosocially constructed identities).

I understand that something must have happened dynamically that analyst and patient later came to understand as a racialized enactment. Yes, that makes a lot of sense. But were the racial stereotypes unconscious? If we employ a Freudian vocabulary, we would say they belong in the realm of the preconscious. I do not put into question that in reenactments of racism, sexism, and classism we are dealing with enactments of something motivated unconsciously, *but* I do not think that we can ever fully capture *it*.

Yet, we are pulled toward the belief and relief that we actually could get there, as in "HA! There we have it. We both participated in re-enacting a racist power dynamic. And now we're good." Not only as in now, in a session, we get to collude less and bring to light more of what lies 'underneath' or 'beyond' those racialized fantasies but also as in, "now, *we* are good, as in, 'us psychoanalysts' who reflect upon racism." We might be tempted by the idea that we could find the good, completely non-harmful way of relating in the world—and that itself may still be influenced by the very tendencies we are trying to overcome. (I am thinking of examples of enforced political correctness—when we call out a person for being racist while at the same time disavowing our own racism.)

And I want to quote Layton in her clinical example in which she is grappling with this dilemma:

> Once I realized that I was performing 'whiteness' to his [the patient's] inferior non-whiteness, I began to ask different questions of him than I had been asking. I tried then to deconstruct whiteness by helping him think about the vulnerable parts of himself that he hated, and how whiteness had both wounded him and become for him a fantasy guarantee that he would never again feel the pain of inferiority and humiliation.

Layton writes:

> I came to recognize that my own pretense to incarnating whiteness is precisely the kind of normative unconscious process that sustains racial inequality. My 'wish' to occupy the position of what I would call 'invulnerability' (rather than wholeness), … demonstrates that racism and class inequality do not only split the psyche of the subordinate; they also bolster the fantasmatic position of the dominant—and *both* parties want to hold to the fantasy that

(as Lacan might say, *someone* has the phallus) "someone is invulnerable to pain and loss."

Conclusion

So, why do I think it's relevant for both psychoanalytic theorizing and clinical work to maintain a notion of 'the unconscious'?

First of all, what we are trying to do is not just a narcissistically motivated exercise of holding up the holy grail of psychoanalysis. Instead, the whole enterprise started with trying to understand stuff that we cannot understand without the supposition of a dynamic unconscious: from dreams, to slips of the tongue, and to so-called symptoms (I am saying so-called because with Erich Fromm I would like to hold the idea of "pathology of normalcy" (Fromm, 1973, p. 356) and not just call symptoms whatever does not fit the current consensus), to the utmost human destructiveness, basically whatever resists rational reasoning and lies at the bottom of racism, sexism, and classism. There always remains a surplus that cannot be grasped without the supposition of 'the unconscious': the fascination that we can have for something horrific, the pleasure that humans can feel when torturing somebody or brutally murdering people, be it in homicides or genocides.

It is the crazy bits of what it means to be human and that reach beyond or beneath the logic of the reproduction of normative identities. If we give up the notion 'the unconscious' in favor of 'unconscious processes,' we might lose the idea of 'a dynamic unconscious.' Since with Freud (1905) and Laplanche (2011), this concept implies a sexual polymorphously perverse unconscious, we might lose out of sight or out of grip the very pleasures and horrors that make up relationships of power, violence, and domination. And I would like to add that whenever we let ourselves be truly affected by that stuff—it tends to be unbearable.

References

Freud, S. (1905). Three essays on the theory of sexuality (1905). In *The standard edition of the complete psychological works of Sigmund Freud*, Volume VII (1901–1905): A case of hysteria, three essays on sexuality and other works (pp. 123–246). (J. Strachey, trans.). London: Hogarth Press.

Fromm, E. (1973). *The anatomy of human destructiveness*. New York, NY: Holt, Rinehart and Winston.

Kubie, L. S. (1974; repr. 2011). The drive to become both sexes. *Psychoanalytic Quarterly, 80*(2), 369–440.

Laplanche, J. (2011). Gender, sex, and the sexual. In *Freud and the sexual: Essays 2000–2006* (pp. 159–190). New York, NY: The Unconscious in Translation.

Part III

Language, the sexual, and the unconscious

Chapter 6

Introduction to a Lacivanian idiolect

Pascal Sauvayre and Orsi Hunyady

Introduction

This chapter comprises a study in comparative psychoanalysis between Lacan and Sullivan on the concept of the unconscious, a study which is riddled with difficulties.

First, the unconscious is fundamentally elusive and slippery, both clinically and theoretically. It gave Freud fits, and Lacan is the first to recognize this difficulty, but rather than backing off from it, he exhorts us to embrace it with him.

> Let's read the texts: let's follow Freud's thought in the detours it imposes on us, and let's not forget that in deploring them himself with respect to an ideal scientific discourse, he affirms that he was forced into them by his object.[1]
>
> (1966, p. 620)

That is, the unconscious.

But this exhortation comes with a warning. Indeed, if the foundational object of psychoanalysis is so slippery, then there is no sense trying to grasp it, to seize it, and even to understand it. This guides his writing, "my *Écrits*, I did not write them in order for people to understand them"[2] (2005, pp. 84–85); instead, he asks his reader to "mettre du sien,"(1966, p. 10), which literally means to 'put of yourself into it.' To convey the effort demanded, this can be translated as 'putting your back into it.' Indeed, he recognizes that his readers must 'work' his writings to the point that they may "wear themselves out"[3] (2005, p. 85); even if validating, this may come as little relief to the reader who has slogged through his writings and been left in a state of total confusion. He continues, "they [the readers] don't understand anything, that is absolutely true, for a while, but it has an impact on them"[4] (2005, p. 85). It is perhaps best to think of the reader in the same position of the patient when Lacan explains that "analytic interpretation is not designed to be understood, it is designed to make waves" (1976, p. 35).

To add to this basic state of confusion, there is the further matter of how they respectively deal with foundational Freudian terms. Sullivan rejects them altogether. He comments, "I tried to say nothing about the unconscious except to suggest that it was not phenomenologically describable. I don't use the conception particularly" (1964, p. 221). Indeed, in his major theoretical work, *The Interpersonal Theory of Psychiatry*, the term does not appear as such. In contrast, Lacan, championing a 'return to Freud,' meticulously retains and expands the Freudian terms throughout his oeuvre. And in *The Four Fundamental Concepts of Psychoanalysis*, the first to be addressed is, the unconscious.

Finally, to punctuate these warnings, Sullivan notes, "it has been so many years since I found anything but headaches in trying to discover parallels between various theoretical systems that I have left that for the diligent and scholarly, neither of which includes me" (1953, p. 167, ff.).

It is therefore with a shaken confidence that we insist that this is a worthwhile endeavor. We propose that an exploration of the widely differing psychoanalytic grammars and vocabularies is an exploration of the richness of psychoanalytic dialogue itself, a richness that is, in our opinion, generated by the slipperiness of its concepts.

These differing grammars and vocabularies, akin to dialects of a common psychoanalytic language, are referred to as idiolects. Moving from one idiolect to the other—and to the best of our knowledge, this has not been attempted yet between these two major thinkers—presents what we would refer to as the 'challenge of translation,' the difficulties of which reach far beyond a straightforward transposition from one idiolect to another. With other languages come other cultures: distinct sensitivities, emphases, attunements, and normative behaviors. A straightforward transposition invariably ends up reducing one language to the other, and results in impoverishment. Instead, a good translation requires a fair amount of interpretation, and a good interpretation is expansive, not reductive; it requires the working over, or better yet the 'working through,' of the terms.

This 'work' exercises the mental muscle of otherness, and how better than to do it through the concept of alterity par excellence, the unconscious.

Lacan's unconscious

Perhaps the best known of Lacan's pithy and obtuse sayings is, "the unconscious is structured like a language"[5] (1973, p. 28). The sentence is tantalizingly simple, even simplistic. It can easily be heard as 'the unconscious is a language.' If that were the case, all we need do is find the Rosetta Stone of the unconscious.

Instead, the key word is the conjunction 'like.' Far from being a conventional language that conveys meaning clearly, "the unconscious is the evasive," Lacan explains, "but we can grasp its outlines within a structure"[6] (1973, p. 41). What then does he mean by structure, and how does it 'outline' the unconscious?

Nature's signifiers

Let's follow Lacan's own example of being awoken out of a nap by a persistent knock at the door. He finally awakens when

> I become conscious of them (the knocks) inasmuch as I reconstitute my entire representation. I know that I am here, at what time I went to sleep, and what I was seeking through this sleep. When the sounds of the knocking reaches, not my perception but my conscious, my conscious reconstitutes itself around that representation.[7]
>
> (1973, p. 66)

What interests him is the period before his awakening, during which the knocks have clearly been perceived and processed into his sleep, ostensibly into a dream. The knocks were perceived, just not consciously. It is in this post-perceptual but pre-consciousness space where we find the outlines of the unconscious.

Grounded in contrast, perception requires a rudimentary structure, so the unconscious should not be confused with a pre-perceptual undifferentiated mass that the cauldron metaphor is often used to represent the id. In order to perceive the knocks, differentiation and opposition between figure and ground, and among figures, are necessary. We are still far from the discrete blocks from which language symbols are constructed, but we can see here that all of the elements of language including letters, syllables, words, and so forth, also require this base oppositional structure. "Even before relations that can be properly called human are established … [there are] themes of opposition. Nature provides, to say the word, signifiers, and these signifiers organize human interactions in inaugural fashion, gives them structures, and models them"[8] (1973, p. 28). The knocks, then, are examples of 'nature's signifiers,' which are differentiated perceptions from which will be mined the signifiers to be used for signification. "Discontinuity, this is thus the essential form in which the unconscious first[9] appears to us as a phenomenon"[10] (1973, p. 34).

Between perception and consciousness

How then do these perceptions, nature's signifiers, become signifiers that generate signification? Let's imagine that Lacan was dreaming of being a prisoner in solitary confinement. He hears knocks on the wall, so he tries to communicate with the other prisoner with his own knocks. Soon enough, using even a random chunking of the knocks, knock knock beat knock beat knock knock beat etc., identifiable patterns will begin to emerge. The combinatory game of the knocks is not yet a language that our prisoners can use to communicate specific meanings, but we can see that it is a language in wait. Each prisoner recognizes the patterns but these remain mysterious, perceived and recognized on one hand, but opaque and enigmatic on the other.

According to Lacan, the building blocks of language emerge out of very simple combinatorial rules that operate on their own; it is 'on top' of these combinatorial rules that the meaning, and the hiding of it, is eventually layered. "The combinatorial game operating in its spontaneity, on its own, in a presubjective way—it is this structure that gives its status to the unconscious"[11] (1973, p. 28).

We should note here that the linguistic nature of Lacan's unconscious makes it fundamentally intersubjective. Each of our prisoners' knocking patterns are blind, yet pregnant, to meaning. There are no reliable signifier-signified connections established yet, so we can imagine both of them in a mad parataxic interpersonal exchange.

In this example, we can see in the unconscious the operation of recognizable perceptual combinations, requiring the activity of the 'other' to move from their 'unformulated' to their 'formulated' states. The term 'unformulated' (which might be familiar to us here) speaks directly to Lacan's concept of the unconscious as structured but unrealized, or of the unformulated in wait of formulation. "The unconscious is manifested to us as something that holds itself in suspense in the area, I would say, of the *unborn*," (1973, p. 23)—i.e., the unrealized, or unformulated, which is quite different from undifferentiated. The unconscious operates "in a register that is neither of the unreal, nor of the derealized, but of the non-realized, ... a larval zone"[12] (1973, p. 31). If we go back to Lacan's knocks, the unconscious 'holds itself in suspense' by 'taking up the knocks' in its own mental activities and by using them as dream material (primary process). If you will, the unconscious gets 'first pick' of what perceptions it will use.

This mental activity can be referred to as "primary process—which is nothing other," Lacan says, "than what I have been trying to define for you in the form of the unconscious, we must ... grasp it in its experience of rupture, between perception and consciousness"[13] (1973, p. 66). This unconscious netherworld between perception and consciousness is called a "béance" (1973, p. 25), often translated as gap. But a more accurate term is 'gaping,' which implies the presence of active forces, necessary to 'hold itself in suspense.' Hence, 'gaping' is a gap that has been actively opened and is being kept open. In French 'béance' also has a medical meaning and refers to an opening in the body maintained by its structure, such as the larynx or trachea, requiring forces to keep it open. Were it not for the structure, the forces would collapse, and the opening would close. The opening can be covered over (as in repression), or controlled (as in censorship), and that allows in/out exchanges between parts of the psyche.

Refinding subjectivity

Up to now, we have been following the transformation of the raw material of perception into conscious meaning, from knocking sounds to knocks at the door. Let's now sit in the seat of Lacan's conscious mind going 'backward.' He realizes that what are now knocks at the door 'were' once dream elements. From the perspective of consciousness, then, this realization is a 'finding'—as in, these knocks at the door were once knocks on the prison wall of my dream. He says, "what is produced in this gaping, in the full sense of the term to produce, presents itself as a find. It is thus that the

Freudian exploration first encounters what occurs in the unconscious"[14] (1973, p. 33).

He goes on: the find is "*the surprise*—that by which the subject feels out of her depth, that by which she finds simultaneously more and less than she was expecting"[15] (1973, p. 33). However, "this find, as soon as it presents itself, is a re-finding, it is always at the ready to steal itself away again, establishing the dimension of the loss"[16] (1973, p. 33). From the perspective of the conscious self, the dream content is a find—something novel, but from the perspective of one's overall subjectivity, it is a refinding of what has remained unrealized.

Lacan reformulates Freud's 'making the unconscious conscious.' Dismissing as "trash" (1973, p. 53) the conventional translations of Freud's, 'wo es war, soll ich werden,' he stays close to the original. 'Where it was, I shall become,' or conversely, 'I shall become where it was' captures better how the subject, the I (not the ego), 'finds' itself where it (not the id) always was, in wait of being (found), it is a refinding of itself in the larval zone.

In other words, if we think of the ego as the crystallization of Lacan's conscious representations of his experience, of himself, it uses the knocks at the door to reconstitute itself, and it relegates the knocks on the prison wall at first to being 'just a dream,' and then they are forgotten. It stands in the way of the movement toward its unrealized origins. "The ego (le moi), in our experience, represents the center of all the resistances,"[17] (1966, p. 118), so "it is indeed in the desegregation of the imaginary unity of the ego that the subject finds [its] signifying material"[18] (1966, p. 427). Refinding subjectivity is therefore not a question of the ego establishing itself on firm ground. Quite the contrary, the subject re-finds itself in an indeterminate, but not undifferentiated, place of its origins—at first the knocks of the prison wall, and further back the knocking sounds, and so on in a regressive direction.

The navel of the unknown

Lacan writes:

> We aim at subjects, and to touch them at what Freud calls the navel—
> the navel of the dream, he writes, to designate in ultimate terms, the
> core of the unknown—which is nothing but, just as the anatomical
> navel that it represents, the gaping which we have referred to.
>
> (1973, p. 31)

The regressive movement aims, in Freud's words, at a "spot in every dream ... which ... is unplumbable—a navel, as it were, that is its point of contact with the unknown"[19] (1900, p. 111 ff.).

If Lacan follows the regressive 'royal road' of the knocks, they will lead him to 'become' where his subjectivity 'was,' and eventually to the origins of his subjectivity—the bottomlessness of the unknown. "Where is the bottom? Is it absence? No. The rupture, the cleft, the stroke of the opening makes absence surge forth—not like the cry taking its shape against a ground of silence but on the contrary as silence"[20] (1976, p. 34).

The lack is not to be confused with nothingness, just as silence is not to be confused with inert absence of sound. It is an absence that 'surges forth'—pushing to the surface the knocks as conveyors of experience that has remained unformulated, unrealized. The unconscious can be said to speak, in a manner of speaking. It is indeed structured like a language.

> At the level of the unconscious there is something at all points homologous with what occurs at the level of the subject—it speaks, it functions in a way that is as elaborate as it is at the level of the conscious, which thus loses what seemed to be its privilege.[21]
>
> (1976, p. 33)

The juncture with the real

This odd language of the unconscious speaks for what is unplumbable, unknowable, and for 'what ultimately lies beyond language itself.' Conventional language spoken by our conscious says only what is already known, hence it doesn't ever say much of anything; 'unconscious language' speaks for what is unformulated, for what evades attempts to 'grasp' it, to 'formulate it.'

What is this 'it'? If we go back to the knocks, we will remember that the unconscious has already 'taken possession' of them as signifiers for the purposes of the dream, so we would expect the dream to continue preserving sleep, and the question becomes: why wake up at all? Lacan answers this by switching to one of Freud's dreams. Here, a father is awakened by fire when "the wrappings and one of the arms of his beloved child's dead body had been burned by a lighted candle that had fallen on them" (1900, pp. 509–510). Lacan surmises that the father awoke not because of the 'reality' of the fire, but because of what he calls the 'real' that the dream was taking him to. The dream had already appropriated nature's signifier of the actual fire and had rendered it into an already atrocious vision: "*his child was standing beside his bed, caught him by the arm and whispered to him reproachfully: 'father don't you see I'm burning?'*" (1900, p. 509). What disturbed the father from his sleep, what did the sleeper escape by waking up? Lacan surmises it was the "beyond" that this atrocious vision of the dream was pointing to: a 'real' that was too much to bear, so the dreamer awoke to reality.

> The waking, how not to see its double meaning—that the waking that locates us back in a constituted and represented reality has a double function? The real, it's beyond the dream that we must search for it— in what the dream has coated, has enveloped, has hidden from us, behind the lack of representation of which there is nothing but a space holder. This is the real that commands our activities more than anything, and it is psychoanalysis that designates them.[22]
>
> (1973, p. 71)

The real is what we are connected to through the navel of the dream. As Lacan conceptualizes it, the unconscious is at the juncture of what cannot be structured, of what negates any psychic organization, what he calls the real. We can then understand that "the real presented itself in the form of something in itself that is *inassimilable*—in the form of trauma, determining all of its developments"[23] (1973, p. 65, italics in the original). Both dream and fantasies are then conceptualized as screens that simultaneously represent and keep at bay the beyond of the real.

Anxiety

The kind of experiences that are exclusive to this domain, such as atrocious visions, are what Sullivan would locate in the register of uncanny emotions. For Lacan, it is at this juncture that we find anxiety.

> Anxiety is for analysis a crucial reference, because indeed anxiety is what does not deceive. In experience, it is necessary to channel it, and if I dare say, to dose it out, if one is not to be submerged by it. It is the correlative difficulty of the one that comes from conjoining the subject with the real.[24]
>
> (1973, p. 49–50)

As what 'does not deceive,' anxiety is therefore fully 'real,' yet it must be filtered, dosed, and in fact distorted, in order to be 'assimilable' to the subject to any degree. Anxiety in the raw of the real simply submerges the subject, like a "blow to the head"—a pivotal metaphor that Sullivan uses on several occasions (for instance, 1953, p. 152 and p. 205).

As the meeting point of the subject and the real, anxiety can also be seen as a meeting point between Lacan and Sullivan.

Sullivan's anxiety

Sullivan opens his book *The Interpersonal Theory of Psychiatry* with the following:

> Insofar as you grasp the concept of anxiety as I shall be struggling to lay it before you, I believe you will be able to follow, with reasonable success, the rest of this system of psychiatry. Insofar as I fail to get across to you the meaning of anxiety, insofar as you presume that I mean just what you now think what anxiety is, I shall have failed to communicate my ideas.
>
> (1953, p. 8)

Given how important it is for him, it is noteworthy that one of anxiety's most important characteristics is its elusiveness, both experientially and theoretically. Initially 'induced' into the infant by the mothering one, anxiety is associated with a sort of dread that calls for immediate action; but in contrast to needs that can be met, anxiety is, given its 'alien' nature (originating in the mother), vague and diffuse and is not associated with any one 'zone of interaction' that would allow the infant to anticipate it or to dissipate it. "Because there is a lack of differentiation in terms of the direction toward its relief by appropriate action, anxiety is not manageable," Sullivan goes on (1953, p. 43).

Instead of anxiety itself being 'managed,' processed, or transformed, only the approach of anxiety can be anticipated through an elaboration of 'signs' ('forbidding gestures' for example) that 'indicate' its presence: "discomfort, tense discomfort, a definite transition from bad to worse, a feeling of general ill-being, all of these are of a single genus—they indicate anxiety" (1970, p. 103). The presence of anxiety is in no way 'grasped' or contained by the mental apparatus, which is in fact devoted to its avoidance, to its negation if you will.

We are suggesting that by virtue of its slipperiness both as concept and as formulatable experience, it is in anxiety, rather than 'covert operations,' that we will find a more robust corollary in Sullivan's theory to the concept of the unconscious.

The prototaxic mode and nature's signifiers

Coming before the ability to organize stimuli into signals, signs, and then symbols, Sullivan refers to the most basic mode of experience as the prototaxic. It is as if "everything that is sensitive and centrally represented were an indefinite, but very greatly abundant, luminous switchboard; and the pattern of light which would show on the switchboard in a discrete experience is the basic prototaxic experience itself" (1953, p. 29). Referred to as "sentience" (1953, p. 29) at this level, the operation of the psyche is organized around contrast and change, or discontinuity as Lacan emphasized, such that the knocking sounds are among the points of lights on the luminous switchboard. They are not yet even strung together as a pattern, but they are perceived as discrete (and therefore differentiated) elements that reflect and thereby constitute a rudimentary structure. In sum, the luminous switchboard can be thought of as providing the necessary level of differentiation and structure to supply the psyche with nature's signifiers. No actual meaning is shaped out of the sensations, but sentience serves as the constituting elements for meanings yet to come.

Severe anxiety and the real

Let's say that there is one bulb on the switchboard so powerful that it drowns out all the others, one 1,000-watt bulb that cancels out the other 20- to 60-watt bulbs—that's the anxiety bulb, turned on and off completely unpredictably by the mother's own anxiety. How does the mother turn it on and off so? Sullivan says, we do not have a clear understanding of the "thoroughly obscure" mechanism that allows for this, but we can "bridge the gap simply by referring to it as a manifestation of an indefinite—that is, not yet defined—interpersonal process to which I apply the term empathy" (1953, p. 41). Empathy allows anxiety in through a direct connection with the mother—a metaphorical umbilical cord.

When the mother's anxiety first invades ("induced in" 1953, p. 53) the infant, it has the effect of a "blow to the head" (e.g., 1953, p. 152), a metaphor that Sullivan uses repeatedly. Shall we say: it knocks the infant out. The remnants of these traumatic instances live on in what we termed uncanny emotions earlier, which possess the shape of feelings but ultimately point back at what is before verbalization and elaboration. They point to Lacan's real; they have "a sort of shuddery, not-of-this-earth component"—to use Sullivan's words—they are "a curious survival from a very early emotional experience," (1953, p. 10) the real of anxiety one could say.

Maybe the purest form in which these early experiences of raw anxiety are preserved later in life are night terrors, where "one awakens from some utterly unknown events in practically primordial terror; in this state, one is on the border of complete disintegration of personality" (1953, p. 334). We can think here of Freud's patient waking up in order to avoid the 'surging forth' of this kind of experience. Awakening closes up the gaping, what we called the navel of the dream, the remainder of the umbilical cord, through which we received the unknowable and intolerable dread that we try forever to make sense of and that stays in the unreachable center of our creative mental endeavors.

The parataxic mode and signification

However unmanageable it may be, anxiety is the developmental motor that brings about the formulation of language, of communication, and of course miscommunication. Beginning not as representations of anxiety, but as we saw, as "signs that indicate its presence," these signs can then become signs of other signs, then organized into symbols, and eventually into somewhat cohesive representational patterns of interpersonal behavior such as good-me and bad-me. The development of signs, symbols, and personifications "elevates complexity or elaboration of experience from the prototaxic mode to the parataxic mode" (1953, p. 84). We should note that this increasing complexity is not a process of incremental approximations of 'reality,' of what actually is, but quite to the contrary, it can be seen as a process of incremental complexity of the avoidance of the 'real of anxiety,' to mix vocabularies. What ultimately cannot be assimilated, prehended, or in any way included in these personifications—even in the form of distortions—can be thought of as making up the remainder, the much vaster land of not-me experiences.

In a passage worthy of Lacan's ambiguity, Sullivan writes, "from the very beginning the potent influence of anxiety permits the organization of experience [and] prevents the organization of experience" (1953, p. 186). At first, this organization is the idiosyncratic culture of the mother-infant dyad and their quasi automatic ('covert') anxiety avoidance maneuvers. For instance, the knocks may have been linked to a traumatic repressed memory of Lacan's mother that she then conveyed to him. The knocks were then a signal of something obscure, uncanny, lying in wait behind the door, as was Lacan. These signs can be said to have proto-meanings, that can only become meanings when co-constructed and consensually validated. However, the fact that we develop the intellectual capacity to 'think' (in the full sense of the word, as performing the work of metaphor) should not be taken as the new purpose of our mental activity, as something that we strive for for its own sake; it is still 'driven,' if you will, and encased by its service to our basic endeavor of "minimizing anxiety."

Back to the navel of the dream

As the parataxic and then the syntactic mode of experiencing emerge, anxiety exists in more 'distant' forms, in gradients. With thinking come dreams and nightmares, which, in contradistinction to the night terrors we mentioned earlier, have recollectable, and formulatable, content. So, they serve as the screen that both separates us from, and connects us to, the 'real of anxiety'—the unassimilable that lies 'beyond.'

Sullivan describes a dream of his own that demonstrates this point. He starts by saying that in infancy he developed an immense, almost unmanageable fear of spiders, which (in his opinion) reflected his relationship to his mother's anxiety. Then he goes on to the dream that he had as an adult: in the dream he notices and then observes beautifully woven geometric patterns on the grass ahead of him, the kind that spiders make, and he follows the patterns because they remind him of textiles—something he is "noticeably interested in," as he points out. Soon, the textile patterns turn into a tunnel (the umbilical cord), and in the tunnel a spider approaches him, slowly gaining horrendous proportions (the navel of the dream). Sullivan is awakened from the dream at this point, but is unable to obliterate the spider from his conscious mind, which he continues to see in the form of a dark spot on the sheet. It is only once he is fully awoken, has gotten out of bed, and performed some unrelated activities, (that he reconstitutes himself, as Lacan does around the knocks of his conscious) that he is able to go back to the bed to inspect the sheet, at which point the spot is gone, and so he deems it safe to go back to sleep (1953, p. 335–336).

Note the radical change that took place in the dream in terms of the movement of the experience itself, such that the curiosity, that initially leads Sullivan down a dangerous path, gave way to fear and a sense of inescapability of this fear, as the dream leads 'him' 'back' to the original dread, touching on the real of anxiety. And like Lacan, and Freud's patient, it is at this point that he awakens to 'reality' to escape the real.

The syntactic mode and the unconscious as a gap

As we saw, Sullivan avoids the term the unconscious, so all the more surprising is his unequivocal endorsement of it in his paper, entitled "The Illusion of Personal Individuality," a title we can imagine Lacan using. "The unconscious … is that which cannot be experienced directly, which fills all the gaps in the mental life; [it] explains the discontinuity in conscious life" (1964, p. 204)—the same gaps, or should we say gapings that are "bridge[d]" by "empathy," which can be seen more as an affliction that mysteriously jumps the gap not from perception to meaning, but rather from perception to its misformulation, at best.

While Lacan looks for these 'béances' mostly in parapraxes, Sullivan is attuned to disruptions, pauses, inconsistencies in the tone and rhythm of the patient's speech and presentation, posture, body language, etc. These gapings are a clear indicator of anxiety 'surging forth,' so it is at these moments that the self-system is on highest alert. "The operations of the self-system are always in opposition to achieving the purpose of the interview," (1970, p. 99) just as the ego 'represents the center of all resistances' for Lacan. But, as the self-system's maneuvers are exposed by the 'expert' participant-observer, "the remarkable aspects of the self-system is that after suffering defeat it immediately pulls itself together and goes to work again," (1970, p. 99) closing the gap.

What do we do to listen for what surges forth? Sullivan has a clear idea of the interviewer as 'expert,' the expert who can find that right balance between too much and too little anxiety, and find the tracks that anxiety has left behind and that the patient's self-system tries to cover up. But the 'expertise' of the clinician is of course riddled with difficulties. As a "participant," the interviewer's self-system adds to the mess, "for the interviewer is not engaged in being anything like a well-rounded person whose durable characteristics would be pertinent to the interview." Hence, "the interviewer is getting in his own way" (1970, p. 97). How do we deal with this predicament?

Clinical applications: The expert as hollowed out analyst

Where does the interviewer get her 'expertise' from? Or, how does she 'find' her expertise? While Sullivan doesn't theorize this matter much at all, Lacan is not hesitant to offer suggestions.

The general principle is that the analyst should 'absent' herself, or rather absent her ego, her 'self-system.' Lacan goes so far as to say that the analyst should "cadaverize" herself, by which he means for her not to speak from the position of her ego. It is not a question of simply being silent, but rather of being present through absence. What are the knocks or the spider saying? Where are they coming from? The analyst's ego, her self-system, stand in the way of listening. When the Lacanian analyst speaks (provides an interpretation), it is not because the analyst has understood, nor is it to be understood by the patient (understanding takes place in the register of the ego, and hence is a 'méconnaissance,' just like the self-system can only lead to a parataxic distortion), but it is to evoke (just like Lacan the author), to make the patient/reader 'work.' Hence Lacan's concept of the enigmatic interpretation, not the correct interpretation but an enigmatic one, makes the patient (not the patient's ego, but the patient's subjectivity) work.

When the ego/self-system loses its prominence, particularly in the analyst, then the road is cleared for the analyst to say something that might trigger actual 'work.' Let's see if we find some of these principles at work in the following exchange.

Sullivan and the patient seem to have reached an impasse in the session, so he suggests an 'experiment':

S: Let us try an experiment and now let us be very candid—will you tell me something about myself? We are trying a practical test.
P: Well, your manner has seemed to be rather affected … especially your enunciation and manner of treating patients. … I have often wondered why it is [that] you have never married … and then I tried to … find some association between your choice of work and the reasons you

have never married—your professional manner didn't seem affected but I had an intuition that it was the result of some effort anyway. And you seem to be under some strain—that is about all, I think.

This is followed by an interaction in which the patient, with Sullivan's encouragement, fleshes out in detail his impressions of Sullivan. Instead of responding to the reality of these impressions, he concludes this exchange thus:

S: if to avoid argument you should be interested in your characterization of me—do you remember it well? Because if you don't, I will be glad to give you a copy of it. It would be … more illuminating than anything else you have said (in Wake, 2011, pp. 39–41).

What an enigmatic place to leave the patient! A Lacanian analyst might have used that moment to end the session, to 'scand' the session so as to punctuate the moments of potential work. And so, we end here.

Notes

1 Lisons les textes: suivons la pensée de Freud en ces détours qu'elle nous impose et dont n'oublions pas qu'en les déplorant lui-même au regard d'un idéal du discours scientifique, il affirme qu'il y fut forcé par son objet.
2 Mes *Écrits*, je ne les ai pas écrits pour qu'on les comprenne.
3 s'esquintent.
4 Ils n'y comprenne rien, c'est tout à fait vrai, pendant un certain temps, mais ça leur fait quelque chose.
5 L'inconscient est structuré comme un language.
6 L'inconscient c'est l'évasif—mais nous arrivons à le cerner dans une structure.
7 J'en (des coups) prends conscience, c'est pour autant qu'autour d'eux, je reconstitue toute ma représentation. Je sais que je suis là, à quelle heure je me suis endormi, et ce que je cherchais par ce sommeil. Quand le bruit du coup parvient, non point à ma perception mais à ma conscience, c'est que ma conscience se reconstitue autour de cette représentation.
8 Dès avant que des relations s'établissent qui soient proprement humaines, … des thèmes d'opposition. La nature fournit, pour dire le mot, des signifiants, et ces signifiants organisent de façon inaugurante les rapports humains, en donnent les structures, et les modèlent.
9 "First" can be understood as part of a perceptual sequence as well as as falling on the spectrum of a developmental trajectory (as in 'primary').
10 La discontinuité, telle est donc la forme essentielle où nous apparaît d'abord l'inconscient comme phénomène.
11 Le jeu combinatoire opérant dans sa spontanéité, tout seul, d'une façon présubjective—c'est cette structure qui donne son statut à l'inconscient.

12 Dans un registre qui n'est rien d'irréel, ni de dé-réel, mais de non-réalisé, …
zone des larves.

13 Le processus primaire—qui n'est autre que ce que j'ai essayé pour vous de
définir … sous la forme de l'inconscient—il nous faut bien … le saisir dans
son expérience de rupture, entre perception et conscience.

14 Ce qui se produit dans cette béance, au sens plein du terme se produire, se
présente comme la trouvaille. C'est ainsi d'abord que l'exploration freud-
ienne rencontre ce qui se passe dans l'inconscient.

15 *La surprise*—ce par quoi le sujet se sent dépassé, par qui il en trouve à la fois
plus et moins qu'il n'en attendait.

16 Cette trouvaille, dès qu'elle se présente, est retrouvaille, et qui plus est, elle
est toujours prête à se dérober à nouveau, instaurant la dimension de la perte.

17 Le moi, dans notre expérience, représente le centre de toute les résistance à la
cure des symptômes.

18 C'est en effet dans la déségrégation de l'unité imaginaire que constitue le moi,
que le sujet trouve le matériel signifiant de ses symptômes.

19 On vise les sujets, et qu'on les touche à ce que Freud appelle le nombril—
nombril des rêves, écrit-il pour en désigner, au dernier terme, le centre
inconnu—qui n'est point autre chose, comme le nombril anatomique même
qui le représente, que cette béance dont nous parlons.

20 Où est le fond? Est-ce l'absence? Non pas. La rupture, la fente, le trait de
l'ouverture fait surgir l'absence—comme le cri non pas se profile sur fond de
silence, mais au contraire comme silence.

21 Au niveau de l'inconscient il y a quelque chose en tous points homologue
à ce qui se passe au niveau du sujet—ça parle, et ça fonctionne d'une façon
aussi élaborée qu'au niveau du conscient, qui perd ainsi ce qui paraissait son
privilège.

22 L'éveil, comment ne pas voir qu'il est à double sens—que l'éveil qui nous
restitue dans une réalité et représentée fait double emploi? Le réel, c'est au-
delà du rêve que nous avons à le rechercher—dans ce que le rêve a enrobé,
nous a caché, derrière le manque de la représentation dont il n'y a là qu'un
tenant-lieu. C'est le réel qui commande plus que tout autre nos activités, et
c'est la psychanalyse qui nous les désigne.

23 Le réel se soit présenté sous la forme de ce qu'il y a en lui d'inassimilable—
sous la forme de trauma, déterminant toute sa suite.

24 L'angoisse est pour l'analyse un terme de référence crucial, parce qu'en effet
l'angoisse est ce qui ne trompe pas. Mais l'angoisse peut manquer. Dans
l'expérience, il est nécessaire de la canaliser et, si j'ose dire, de la doser, pour
n'en être pas submergé. C'est là une difficulté corrélative de celle qu'il y a à
conjoindre le sujet avec le réel.

References

Freud, S. (1900). *The interpretation of dreams*. The Standard Edition of the
Complete Psychological Works of Sigmund Freud, Volume IV (1900): The
Interpretation of Dreams (First Part), ix–627.
Lacan, J. (1966). *Ecrits*. Paris: Seuil.

Lacan, J. (1973). *Les quatres concepts fondamentaux de la psychanalyse.* Paris: Seuil.

Lacan, J. (1976). *Lectures and conferences at North American universities.* Scilicet 6/7. Paris: Seuil.

Lacan, J. (2005). *Le triomphe de la religion.* Paris: Seuil.

Sullivan, H. S. (1953). *The interpersonal theory of psychiatry.* New York, NY: Norton.

Sullivan, H. S. (1964). *The fusion of psychiatry and the social sciences.* New York, NY: Norton.

Sullivan, H. S. (1970). *The psychiatric interview.* New York, NY: Norton.

Wake, N. (2011) *Private practices: Harry Stack Sullivan, the science of homosexuality, and American liberalism.* New Brunswick, NJ: Rutgers University Press.

ARE LACAN AND SULLIVAN LINKED BY THEIR CONCEPTIONS OF ANXIETY AND THE UNASSIMILABLE? DISCUSSION OF SAUVAYRE AND HUNYADY

Donnel B. Stern

Pascal Sauvayre and Orsi Hunyady have offered us an ingenious interweaving of the theories of the unconscious written by Jacques Lacan and Harry Stack Sullivan. I can't imagine two more unlikely candidates for a comparison of one writer to another—and yet Sauvayre and Hunyady have pulled it off. They have offered us a bridge between continents that have each supported only indigenous life; and therefore, what they have said seems more significant to me than whether I fully agree with it. I do see significant links between the two theories; but I also differ with some of the connections these authors propose, and I will try to say why at the end of my remarks. I admire what they have done, though, because any project that allows 'us' to talk to 'them,' or 'them' to 'us' is a real accomplishment. In fact, any project that allows interpersonal and relational analysts to make any kind of sense of Lacan is a very good thing. I appreciate the authors' fulfillment of their own intellectual aims in this chapter, and their very serious play.

The psychoanalytic theories of North America and France have been virtually incommensurable for a very long time. And if that's true in the general case—that is, if it's true for the psychoanalyses of these two places—it's certainly true in the case of Lacan, who is very French, and Sullivan, who is just as thoroughly American. Despite this situation, though, I have thought for a couple of decades now that a comparison of my own thinking with Lacan's would be a good idea—and apparently, I wasn't the only one to have that thought. In about 1990, at the annual meetings of Division 39 (Psychoanalysis) of the American Psychological Association in Chicago, I served as the discussant on a panel composed of papers on constructivism in psychoanalysis by Louis Fourcher, Irwin Hoffman, and Michael Tansey. During the discussion after I spoke, an older man in the audience stood up and said, with gruffness, even severity, but also with what I thought was a gleam in his eye, "Dr. Stern, could you please tell us the relation of your ideas to those of Jacques Lacan?" There was just the faintest note of amusement in the man's delivery, and I imagined that he knew very well the discomfort his question caused me. Only a very few Americans in those days knew Lacan's work, and I was certainly not one of them. If that's what the man thought—that I would be uncomfortable—he was right. In fact, he was probably even more right than he knew, because, though I didn't yet know him, I did recognize him from book jacket photos. It was Merton Gill, an intellectual hero to me, a man whose work I had read and admired ever since I began in the field of psychoanalysis. Hoping to escape this fix without being humiliated, I said to him, with what I hoped would come out as a humorous edge, "Dr. Gill, I don't know whether to thank you or to kill you!" Thankfully, he seemed to think this was very funny. He sat down, and with the rest of the audience he laughed and laughed. I never had to answer the question.

Even all these years later, although I have learned something about Lacan in the interim, I don't feel in a position to offer a definitive answer to Gill's question—or, for that matter, to comment as expertly as I would like to on what Sauvayre and Hunyady have said. I am still no Lacan expert. But I will do my best.

I know that the chapter you have just read is difficult, especially if you are not already a student of Lacan. So what I intend to do, having had the opportunity to read the chapter several times, is to lay out my understanding of what Sauvayre and Hunyady have said, and to intersperse this review with some commentary of my own.

Why is comparative psychoanalysis so difficult? Sauvayre and Hunyady's thoughts on this matter bear a close relation to my own understanding, which I have written about elsewhere (Stern, 2013). As a matter of fact, in addition to its merit as an outline of commonalities between the work of Lacan and Sullivan, the chapter you've just read is valuable as the presentation of a method of comparative psychoanalysis. One way of reading the chapter, that is, is as the use of the Lacan-Sullivan comparison as an illustration of how to conduct comparative thinking in our field.

After referring to what they call the "diversity and heterogeneity" of psychoanalysis, Sauvayre and Hunyady describe psychoanalysis as also having an underlying unity, like variants of a single language. Each writer's theory is an 'idiolect' (one person's idiosyncratic use of language), of the larger, underlying psychoanalytic discourse. To describe theories as idiolects is to emphasize diversity (each theory's unique purview) within an underlying unity (the broader 'language' that defines psychoanalysis). If theories are idiolects, the authors suggest, it should be possible, within the limits supplied by the uniqueness of each approach, to translate them into one another's terms.

I like this conception, but it brings problems with it, because we must decide from which of the two versions, or idiolects, of psychoanalysis to start; and the starting place then determines which of the two positions is the standard against which the other is defined. Inevitably, then, one dialect or idiolect must be privileged over the other, one set of ideas over the other. When we translate from English to French, for example, we ask—if our native tongue is English—whether some expression in French conveys what we mean by some particular phrase in English. We know that translation is not exact, and so we expect there to be an excess meaning that cannot be contained within the bounds of the comparison. If we are translating from English into French, then we assume that the English version will, by necessity, convey our meaning more completely than the French one. And vice versa, of course: if we begin in French and translate into English, the French version will be more complete. There is a loss of information, so to speak, as there used to be, in the old days before digital recording, when you transferred sound from vinyl records to audiotape, or images from film to videotape.

Presenting the theories of Lacan and Sullivan as if they are interpretations of the same underlying reality, has the effect of draining away the privileging of one theory over another—and perhaps this is part of the reason that Sauvayre and Hunyady embed the differences between the two theories in a larger unity. In a sense, this is what the structuralists did—writers like Levi-Strauss, for instance, or Chomsky—who posited underlying structures in human life, structures that were expressed in different ways in different cultures, but which were nevertheless the same in certain basic respects from one culture to another. Let me quote Sauvayre and Hunyady at some length here. After pointing out that the strength of psychoanalysis is its diversity and heterogeneity, a point with which I agree, Pascal and Orsi write that "an exploration of these different grammars and vocabularies is an exploration of the richness of psychoanalytic dialogue itself." They point out that a comparison of the idiolects of Sullivan and Lacan, and the creation of a single idiolect that contains both, has not been attempted before, and then they write this paragraph, in which they tell us some of what I have just summarized:

> Moving from one idiolect to the other presents what we would refer to as the 'challenge of translation,' the difficulties of which reach far beyond a straightforward transposition from one idiolect to another.

With other languages come other cultures: distinct sensitivities, emphases, attunements, and normative behaviors. A straightforward transposition invariably ends up reducing one language to the other, and results in impoverishment. Instead, a good translation requires a fair amount of interpretation, and a good interpretation is expansive, not reductive; it requires the working over, or better yet the 'working through,' of the terms. This 'work' exercises the mental muscle of otherness, and how better than to do it through the concept of alterity par excellence, the unconscious.

The chapter we have just read is based on this kind of interpretive translation. Let me see if I can describe the nature of this interpretive link. I want to begin with the single, underlying psychoanalytic reality that it seems to me Sauvayre and Hunyady are using as the basis of their theoretical translation: the case they have offered for a relationship between the work of Lacan and Sullivan is rooted in a particular, underlying conception of psychoanalysis that they imply informs both writers.

The paradigm from which Sauvayre and Hunyady are working is, most basically, Freud's (1914) conception of primary narcissism. In Freud's model, the granddaddy of many, if not most, psychoanalytic models of development, the mind begins in an undifferentiated state, with no difference between inside and outside, you and me, before and after, and so on; and development is a matter of the differentiation of discrete structures and functions from this beginning. We see variations on this theme—just for example—in Mahler's (e.g., Mahler, Pine, and Bergman, 1975) description of the symbiotic phase, Loewald's (1951) conception of primary unity, Matte-Blanco's (1988) principle of symmetry, Bion's (1965, 1970) formless infinite—and in Lacan's (1977/2004) understanding of what he called "the real." In development, we see in each of these models the coalescence of more and more differentiated structures from this primal soup: Mahler's baby begins to separate and individuate, developing an ego; in Loewald's scheme the process of interpersonal life leads to formation of more and more sophisticated psychic structures, which eventually reconnect to one another in ways that bring the emotional power of primary unity back into psychic structure; for Matte-Blanco, the differentiating influence of the asymmetrical mode eventually breaks up the infinite sets of the unconscious into discrete meanings; Bion's formless infinite, via projective identification and the sojourn of beta elements in the mother's mind (reverie), becomes alpha elements, allowing the creation of waking dream thoughts. In Lacan's (1977/2004) case, the real is first tamed, in the mirror stage, by the imaginary, and then transformed, as the imaginary is overwritten by the symbolic, into language and thinkable meaning by the name of the father.

I apologize for the brevity of my references to this collection of immense theoretical edifices. What I want to emphasize, though, is not so much the particular contents of each of these models, but the fact that they all have in common, along with many other theories, the principle that the differentiated, adult mind develops from undifferentiated beginnings.

Now, here I think we see an important commonality with Sullivan's scheme of experience. Sullivan's (unfortunately named) prototaxic, parataxic, and syntaxic modes of experience (Sullivan, 1953) are developmental stages that, like Lacan's real, imaginary, and symbolic registers of experience, also become aspects of psychic functioning that continue throughout life. It is also very interesting that for both writers, language is the instrument of this differentiation—it is language, in both schemes, that is, that breaks up the original oneness of experience and makes thought possible. For Lacan, it is the advent of metaphor via the name of the father that ushers in the symbolic and thereby creates the possibility of thought. For Sullivan, it is verbal language that potentiates parataxic experience, which, via consensual validation, becomes syntaxic experience, and thereby thinkable. These notable similarities came about in these two writers' work independently, since it is virtually inconceivable that they could have read one another.

By themselves, these similarities are enough to make the project of comparing Lacan and Sullivan significant and interesting. But they are, in a sense, empirical observations: they don't really require much interpretation, if any. Sauvayre and Hunyady's project is more ambitious than that. It is in the next step of their argument that what they say about the creative, interpretive aspect of translation comes into play. It is in this next step that the writers construct the connection that leads them to claim the existence of a "Lacivanian" idiolect. Let me begin the examination of this major point by quoting another key passage from the chapter:

> As Lacan conceptualizes it, the unconscious is at the juncture of what cannot be structured, of what negates any psychic organization, what he calls the real. We can then understand that "the real presented itself

in the form of something in itself that is *inassimilable*—in the form of trauma, determining all of its developments." Both dream and fantasies are then conceptualized as screens that simultaneously represent and keep at bay the beyond of the real.

Here we have the basis of the combined, Lacivanian idiolect Sauvayre and Hunyady want to suggest to us: the unconscious is the unassimilable. And the unassimilable is the traumatic.

The argument has one last step: the traumatic is captured by the concept and experience of anxiety in both Lacan and Sullivan. It is anxiety that serves as the hinge linking these two theories, and in both cases, anxiety is the sign of inassimilability; it is the sign of trauma. Sauvayre and Hunyady first give us Lacan's version of this argument, beginning with a quotation from Lacan.

Anxiety is for analysis a crucial reference, because indeed anxiety is what does not deceive. In experience, it is necessary to channel it, and if I dare say, to dose it out, if one is not to be submerged by it. It is the correlative difficulty of the one that comes from conjoining the subject with the real.

And then Pascal and Orsi offer this commentary:

As what 'does not deceive,' anxiety is therefore fully 'real,' yet it must be filtered, dosed, and in fact distorted, in order to be 'assimilable' to the subject to any degree. Anxiety in the raw of the real simply submerges the subject, like a "blow to the head."

Like "a blow to the head!" Now we're on familiar ground. We recognize this reference to Sullivan's version of anxiety. Sauvayre and Hunyady focus on what Sullivan called "uncanny emotion" and want us to link it to the kind of experience Lacan refers to when he directs us to Freud's (1900) patient's dream of the burning child. Ingeniously, Sauvayre and Hunyady take Sullivan's (1953, p. 335) famous dream of the spider, also well known to us, as the illustration of this link between the theories. Just as the father in Freud's example wakes from his dream because what would come next would be too horrible, too traumatic, to bear, or even to create in symbolic, knowable form, so Sullivan wakes from his dream of the spider. Sullivan is even more deeply affected than the father of the burning child, though, because after he awakens, he still sees the spider on the bedclothes. It takes several minutes for this little piece of traumatic psychic reality to dissipate.

Sauvayre and Hunyady want us to consider the possibility that the baby takes on the mother's terrible, unconscious anxiety via what Sullivan calls emotional contagion. The prototaxic mode of experience—the most primitive mode—is in this way defined as what is unassimilable, just like Lacan's real. Both the real and prototaxis therefore thoroughly resist any kind of symbolization, while simultaneously serving as an inexhaustible resource for the rest of life; and the rest of life, one might say, is devoted to the attempt to give representation to this material: for Lacan, by the very particular form of representation called the symbolic; for Sullivan, by the parataxic and syntaxic modes of experience.

Now, as I've already said, we know how Sauvayre and Hunyady believe Sullivan's prototaxis is created, and why it is traumatic and unassimilable: it is created via emotional contagion; and this contagion transfers the mothering one's anxiety, which is unbearable, to the baby. Mother's prototaxis becomes baby's prototaxis; mother's anxiety becomes baby's anxiety. But I think Sauvayre and Hunyady haven't really explained the same point in Lacan's theory (or at least in the later versions of Lacan's theory, since Lacan changed his view of the real over time). It hasn't been explained, that is, why the real is defined as originary trauma. I hope Sauvayre and Hunyady explain this in the fuller version of this chapter they will no doubt write. But I don't have a reason to contest this part of their argument.

For the moment, then, I accept that this is a supportable reading of Lacan. On that basis, let's accept the authors' premise: i.e., that anxiety in Lacan's theory can be understood as an expression of the real, and that anxiety in Sullivan's theory can be understood as the expression of prototaxis. If we accept that these readings are viable, what can we say about the connection between the two theories?

I think we can say that drawing this connection is brilliant. I think we can say it's creative and provocative. They have created, or discovered, a single idiolect (their particular discourse of anxiety trauma, and primary unity) within which the two theories can be accommodated; and better than that, this new idiolect makes us think new thoughts about both theories. I hope very much that Sauvayre and Hunyady carry their argument further and that they develop its implications even more fully than the limitations of a single communication have allowed.

But as much as I admire the path these writers have taken in creating this analysis, and as fascinated as I am by their conclusions, I also have some basic questions. Sauvayre and Hunyady make Sullivan sound more like Laplanche than makes sense to me. The idea that prototaxic experience is created by the transfer of the mother's own prototaxic (that is, traumatically anxious) experience, and that the baby then spends its life trying to create a symbolic (in Sullivan's terms, parataxic and syntaxic) form for this unassimilable material, sounds an awful lot like Laplanche's (e.g., 2011) theory that the baby's mind is rooted in the interpretation of the "enigmatic message" implanted in the baby as a byproduct of all of the mothering one's caretaking ministrations. The mother's unconscious anxieties, part of 'the sexual' (which is not to be confused with sexuality per se in Laplanche's thinking), and unknown even to her, are transmitted, without any intention on the mother's part, to the baby, who has no choice but to take them in, and then to be most basically (and unconsciously, like the mother) constituted by them. Laplanche, like Sullivan in the picture offered to us by Sauvayre and Hunyady, claims that the unconscious— portrayed, of course, as the most significant influence on living—is created by the continuous necessity for us to translate and re-translate that mysterious and enigmatic message implanted in the first months of life.

But is this really the meaning of what Sullivan writes? Does this view not do away with Sullivan's entire developmental model? It is certainly true that anxiety lies at the heart of Sullivan's thinking, and that the mind, and experience, are largely shaped by the attempt to evade it. But I think Sullivan's theory of interpersonal relations is about the impact that people have on one another all the way through infancy, childhood, adolescence, and adulthood. The compression of formative events into the very beginning of life is exactly what Sullivan had in mind when he rejected the inevitability of the Oedipus complex and created his views of ongoing interpersonal experience—what Philip Bromberg calls "developmental trauma."

Rather than focusing attention on the ways in which different writers represent a common underlying reality, I would usually rather describe the unique and creative views each writer creates in his or her work. I would usually rather focus my attention, that is, on the worldmaking properties of each psychoanalytic theory, the way each theory constructs its own reality.

That, to me, is what theories are: tools for the construction of worlds; and the success and strength of a theory is therefore to be measured by the extent to which it introduces us to worlds we immediately recognize but never knew before.

But even if I cannot agree with Sauvayre and Hunyady's chapter in certain important respects, I read it with fascination, enthusiasm, and appreciation. I look forward to hearing more about the ideas it contains. This is thinking outside the box; this is scholarship with heart.

References

Bion, W. R. (1965). *Transformations*. London: Heinemann.

Bion, W. R. (1970). *Attention and interpretation*. London: Tavistock Publications.

Freud, S. (1900). *The interpretation of dreams*. The Standard Edition of the Complete Psychological Works of Sigmund Freud, Volume IV (1900): The Interpretation of Dreams (First Part), ix–627.

Freud, S. (1914). *On narcissism*. The Standard Edition of the Complete Psychological Works of Sigmund Freud, Volume XIV (1914–1916): On the History of the Psycho-Analytic Movement, Papers on Metapsychology and Other Works, 67–102.

Lacan, J. (1977/2004). *Ecríts: A selection* (B. Fink, H. Fink, & R. Grigg, Trans.). New York, NY: Norton.

Laplanche, J. (2011). *Freud and the sexual: Essays 2000–2006* (J. House, J. Fletcher, & N. Ray, Trans.). New York, NY: The Unconscious in Translation.

Loewald, H. W. (1951). Ego and reality. *International Journal of Psychoanalysis*, *32*, 10–18.

Mahler, M. S., Pine, F., & Bergman, A. (1975). *The psychological birth of the human infant*. New York, NY: Basic Books.

Matte-Blanco, I. (1988). *Thinking, feeling, and being: Clinical reflections on the fundamental antinomy of human beings and the world*. London and New York, NY: Routledge.

Stern, D. B. (2013). Why is comparative psychoanalysis so difficult? Response to commentaries by Foehl and Troise on "Field theory in psychoanalysis, Part I: Harry Stack Sullivan and Madeleine and Willy Baranger." *Psychoanalytic Dialogues*, *23*, 523–527.

Sullivan, H. S. (1953). *The interpersonal theory of psychiatry*. New York, NY: Norton.

Chapter 7

Après-Coup

Jonathan House

This chapter is based on a talk I gave at the White. The only changes are those required for changing an oral presentation to a written one. The talk extended and refined my papers on après-coup condensing that work by omitting the background, some arguments, and most of the detailed research (2017 and 2015). The major challenge remained unchanged: how to present five interpenetrating concepts in a way that could be followed without pain. I've inserted a handout (Figure 7.1) distributed at the talk: a flow chart showing Laplanche's notion of the origin of the repressed Unconscious. Because I base so much on Laplanche's work, I have also inserted a list I sometimes use as an attempt to present some of Laplanche's key concepts in seven bullet points.

Because the concepts of après-coup and of translation are inextricable, I'll begin with a word on translation, more precisely with Freud's 1896 explanation of repression as a "failure of translation" (1985, p. 208) as the mechanism of the primal repression that creates the Unconscious. (Here it will be helpful to consult Figure 7.1.) Laplanche adopts and extends this translational theory of repression. Primal repression creates the Unconscious and secondary repression is responsible for ongoing additions to the Unconscious. Communications that are successfully translated, that are not repressed, are added to the ego.

Après-coup, Freud's Nachträglichkeit, is an essential psychoanalytic concept—essential but under theorized, and 'under theorized' understates the case. Freud never made it the subject of a paper, his explanations are largely implicit, and his clearest explanations are in his letters

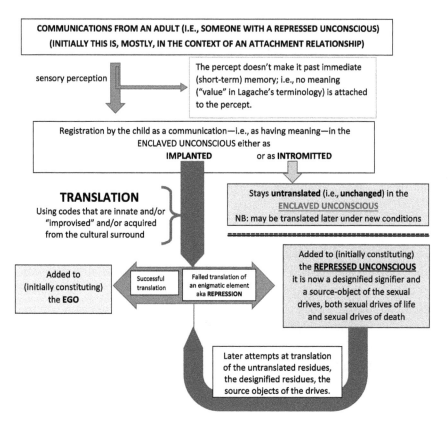

Figure 7.1 Implantation and Intromission of Enigmatic Messages in the Unconscious

to Fliess, which only became available after *The Standard Edition* was almost finished. So, it is no surprise that Strachey's team did not understand the concept and translated the relevant words inconsistently. When they did notice the concept as a concept, they translated it as 'deferred action.' In English, since 1993, the concept has been subjected to the opposite and equally impoverished translation: 'retrospective modification.' Although après-coup is neither deferred action nor retrospective modification, contrasting those two mental processes is useful to providing an explanation.

Deferred action has the temporal structure of fireworks. The beautiful lights in the night sky are the deferred action; they were designed when the device was constructed, designed in the past. *A deferred action is determined by what was desired in the past.*

A retrospective modification is determined by what is desired in the present. It is a story about the past written to meet present needs. A recent example is Donald Trump's retrospective exaggeration of the number of people at his inauguration.

In 1953, Lacan pointed to something noteworthy in Freud's use of the word *nachträglich* and translated it with the two-word phrase '*après-coup.*' Shortly thereafter, the phrase disappeared until 1967 when Laplanche and Pontalis published *The Language of Psychoanalysis*. In their four-page entry (pp. 111–114) on après-coup they write:

> although [Freud] never offered a definition, much less a general theory, of the notion of après-coup, [he] indisputably looked upon [it] as part of his conceptual equipment.

It took another 22 years before après-coup was the object of a major work—Laplanche's lectures of 1989–1990.

When something is hard to understand, Freud recommends that we turn to the poets. I'll turn to *The Odyssey* although Homer only gives the first half of après-coup: après-coup as seduction, as compelling attention.

When, after nine years of pleasant captivity, Odysseus is getting ready to leave Circe's island, the goddess warns him of dangers in his path. The first is a song, the song of the Sirens whose island is littered with corpses of sailors who came close enough to hear the song's seduction. Odysseus blocks the ears of his crew with beeswax and has himself lashed halfway up the mast so that he can hear the song without being lured to his death. Homer allows us to join Odysseus and to hear the song that is impossible to resist. It is only eight lines long. Like many jazz standards, it begins with an intro and then launches into the A section, the seduction, the melody, and the lyrics we remember. Here is the intro:

> Come closer famous Odysseus—Achaea's pride and glory—
> moor your ship on our coast so you can hear our song!
> Never has any sailor passed our shores in his black craft
> until he has heard the honeyed voices pouring from our lips,
> and once he hears to his heart's content sails on, a wiser man.

Now the seduction:

> We know all the wounds that the Greeks and Trojans once endured
> on the spreading plain of Troy when the gods willed it so—
> all that comes to pass on the fertile earth, we know it all![1]

> *That's it!* The Sirens promise a song about wounds, about the
> suffering Greeks and Trojans once endured.

Two points deserve emphasis. First, the seductive story the Sirens offer
Odysseus is his own story. Second, the story is not about victories or
pleasures; it's not about the wily cleverness for which he has been
praised from the opening verse of the epic. The Sirens sing to Odysseus
of suffering; not only of his own suffering, they also sing of the pains
and traumas of others, Greeks and Trojans, friends and enemies. The
irresistible seduction turns out to be the story of suffering experienced
and suffering witnessed. Odysseus is compelled to reminisce. This is a
model for après-coup. Remember the famous sentence from "Preliminary
Communication": "Hysterics suffer mainly from reminiscences" (Breuer
and Freud, 1893).

   Homer does not show the other half of après-coup, what Odysseus does
with the memories, the reminiscing. That's where translation comes in for
the second time. There already was a translation—the assignment of meaning—when Odysseus first witnessed the events; reminiscing provides the
second and later translations. Translation provides a model for après-coup
and for Freud's notion that the mechanism of repression is the failure of
translation which I mentioned earlier. So, let's return to that 1896 letter to
Fliess. Freud is writing to Fliess about memory:

> I should like to emphasize the fact that the successive registrations
> [of memories] represent the psychic achievement of successive
> epochs of life. At the boundary between two such epochs a transla-
> tion of the psychic material must take place. I explain the peculi-
> arities of the [defense] neuroses by supposing that this translation
> has not taken place [for] some of the material, which has certain
> consequences. ... *A failure of translation is known clinically as
> "repression."*
>
> (1985, p. 208, emphasis added)

Repression is a failure of translation, a partial failure, leaving 'some material' untranslated. These untranslated residues constitute the Unconscious and provoke repeated attempts at translation. As will be discussed below, certain residues can never be fully or satisfyingly translated and so will forever demand to be translated and re-translated.

To the extent that translations are determined by the original texts, there is deferred action. To the extent that translators bring something new to the original text, there is retrospective modification. Reminiscing about an event may produce a new translation: the initial understanding of the event, the initial translation, interacts with all subsequent translations of the event to inform the new translation. That new translation is added to conscious/pre-conscious memory, to the ego, while simultaneously the collection of residues in the Unconscious and their interactions are changed.

In addition to the ongoing creation of the Unconscious by repression, après-coup structures psychic trauma and infantile sexuality. To make this clear, we must restore three of Freud's conceptual distinctions that have been obscured, distinctions that are essential to his thinking. Although Freud's terminology is not consistent, the three conceptual distinctions are clear and consistent. They are

- the distinction between psychic trauma and physical trauma
- the distinction between drive and instinct
- the distinction between infantile sexuality and sexuality as a whole

These distinctions have been repressed. Less polemically, one could say that continuity has been emphasized when Freud's contribution was precisely to emphasize the discontinuity. One could call it a failure of translation.

The distinction between psychic trauma and physical trauma

The first step in restoring this distinction is to underline the difference between two kinds of mental processes, each of which involves meaning. Some meaningful mental processes have causes that do not involve meaning: meningitis can cause hallucinations; hyperthyroidism can cause anxiety. To point out that the hallucinations are unrealistic and that the anxiety is irrational is to acknowledge that the hallucinations and the anxiety are meaningful mental events even though their causes are not. In contrast, some meaningful mental events have meaningful mental causes.

Freud's distinction between the psychoneuroses—the neuroses of defense—and actual neuroses makes this conceptual point clear even though his notion that libido is a hormone is silly. The cause of an actual neurosis is physical, bodily: too much or too little libido. The symptoms may be physical or mental or both. In Freud's terminology, hyperthyroidism and febrile delirium are actual neuroses because mental symptoms arise from purely physical causes, that is, from a currently present (actual) condition not caused by thinking.

In contrast, a defense neurosis is caused by thinking, by an occurrence of a mental conflict between "incompatible" ideas. That is how Freud defined psychic trauma. Of course, Freud was a materialist and for him all thinking is instantiated in brain. To say that psychic trauma is "an occurrence of incompatibility" in mental life (1894, p. 47) is not to deny that it is a material event but to say that the material event involves thinking and meaning. While the causes of defense neuroses involve thinking, the symptoms may be physical or mental or both. Thus, the distinction between neuroses of defense and actual neuroses is the distinction between causes that involve meaning and causes that do not.

In *Studies on Hysteria*, Breuer and Freud differed on their understanding of the nature of psychic trauma and also differed on the role and importance both of repression and of sexuality. In brief, Freud thought all hysteria was the result of purposeful repression caused by psychic trauma defined as an incompatibility in mental life that involved sexuality. Breuer thought the creation of unconscious mental contents could be the result of a hypnoid state, that it need not involve motivated repression and still less that sexuality was a requirement. As late as 1895, Freud believed repression was a conscious decision to forget. He gave up that notion, but he never gave up the notion that repression requires incompatible ideas, mental conflict.

To sum up in a phrase, the distinction between physical trauma and 'psychic trauma' is the distinction between stepping on a thumbtack and desiring a forbidden object.

I only have time to emphasize, but not to explain, that until the end of his life, Freud insisted that only what is sexual can be repressed. To make this less counterintuitive, let me remind you that, despite what is sometimes said, Freud explicitly recognized the importance of aggression from the beginning of his work, from the 1890s, and from the beginning explicitly included aggression within sexuality. For instance, in 1905, in the first edition of *Three Essays*, he wrote: "the desire to inflict pain upon the sexual object, and its reverse" is the "most common and the most significant of all the perversions" (1905, p. 219). For Freud, all infantile sexuality is perverse; it always includes sadism and masochism and indeed, at least potentially, all other perversions. What got Freud interested in sexuality was its association with repression, the aggressive sexuality of the perverse adult's traumatogenic sexual approach to a child. Structured by après-coup, the translational theory of repression of 1896 shows why only sexual trauma can lead to repression.

The distinction between instinct and drive

The conflation of instinct and drive has been the bane of psychoanalytic theorizing of sexuality. One reason for the conflation is well known: *The Standard Edition* uses a single word, 'instinct,' to translate two German words, *trieb*, the word for 'drive,' and *instinkt*, the word for 'instinct.' I will skip discussion of these signifiers and go directly to what they signify because the fundamental reason for the conflation is that drive and instinct merge at puberty.

Biologists define instinct like this in the following way. An instinct is an innate, neurological mechanism that, in response to internal or external stimuli, produces actions which contribute to the survival of the individual or of the species.

Some instinctual actions are entirely dependent on physiology: breathing, heart rate, blood pressure, digestion, etc. Such autonomous instincts could be called 'one-person' instincts. Autonomous instincts are sometimes used as a model for all instinctual behavior. This is misleading as some instinctual behavior requires the participation of another human. Remember Winnicott! "There is no such thing as a baby" (1965, p. 39). Limited to one-person instincts, the baby's instinctual repertoire is utterly inadequate for life. A baby's cries communicate with adults and elicit responses necessary for survival. This instinctual call and response falls in the domain of attachment. As Laplanche writes, "attachment is primarily a reciprocal relation of communication and messages" (2000, p. 18).

Before 1897, Freud thought that normally sexuality began at puberty and any sexuality in prepubertal children was created by an adult's sexual approach. This was Freud's seduction theory, an intersubjective under-standing of the origin of hysteria. When he gave up that understanding, he did not abandon the concept of an unconscious; he generalized it. He realized that the Unconscious is universal and thus that every child has an Unconscious. Because Freud did not abandon the notion that the Unconscious is created by the repression of sexuality, it followed that childhood sexuality is also universal. This infantile sexuality is what Freud began to theorize in 1905 in the first edition of *Three Essays on the Theory of Sexuality*. Freud assumed that infantile sexuality is innate and autono-mous, like breathing. Locating the origin of the sexual drives within the individual, he lost sight of the intersubjective.

To be repressed, innate sexuality had to be an idea, one side of an incompatibility of ideas. This led Freud to posit innate ideas, innate sexual fantasies, primal fantasies. Good Darwinist, strict materialist, bench sci-entist, Freud recognized the problems involved in the notion of genetic inheritance of fantasies. But without primal fantasies he would have to abandon infantile sexuality and therefore abandon both repression and the repressed Unconscious.

The concepts needed to explain the origin of infantile sexuality without relying on primal fantasies were not available in Freud's lifetime. In 1987, Laplanche proposed "the general theory of seduction." Later he called the same complex of ideas "the fundamental anthropological situation." This is a model for the origin of infantile sexuality that is not based on the inheritance of ideas. With the general theory of seduction, the problem of the relationship of mind and brain in the theory of the sexual drives no longer needs to be placed on the Procrustean bed of instinct nor fudged and covered up as Freud did with phrases like "frontier" concept and with metaphors that put a ghost in the machine such as "psychical representa-tive" and "the demand made upon the mind for work" (for instance, 1905, p. 168). It also avoids the alchemy of Kleinians who transmute mundane physiologic functions like eating into structuring sexual phantasies—the power of their sorcery is made evident by transforming fantasy's leaden f into a golden ph.

Beyond the question of their origin, Freud recognized two major differ-ences between instincts and drives. Within this chapter, there is only space to name and briefly to specify these differences. The economics and the objects of drives and instincts are radically different.

- *Economics*: The self-preservative instincts of all living entities, from plants to humans, are structured by homeostasis; instincts maintain a stable internal state. In contrast, sexual drives are characterized by the pursuit of increasing and unstable excitation.
- *Objects*: The object of each instinct is specific. Food cannot replace air as the object of the respiratory instinct. In contrast, the objects of the sexual drives are polymorphous and fungible.

The distinction between infantile sexuality and sexuality as a whole

Before turning to après-coup, we must undo a third conflation, the conflation of infantile sexuality with sexuality as a whole. One way to approach this problem is to ask how the attachment system is related to infantile sexuality. Freud opened up this question by identifying a key distinction. Freud dealt with attachment under the rubric of 'self-preservation,' sometimes calling it the tender or "affectionate current" (1905, p. 200). He saw a fundamental opposition between self-preservative or "tender' urges on the one hand and sexual urges on the other. Remember the structure of *Three Essays*. In the first essay, Freud shows that human sexuality is polymorphous and not limited to behavior "contributing to the survival of the individual or of the species," in other words, sexuality is different from instinctual behavior.

Nowadays, there is general agreement that at least some aspects of adult sexuality are not innate but learned, constructed. There is less agreement about infantile sexuality. Like Freud, some colleagues cannot conceive of infantile sexuality except as innate and so conflate it with appetitive urges; others focus on behavioral correlates of biological sex like rough and tumble play. These goings-astray can be blamed on Freud's contradictory and confused theorizing. Notably, the final versions of *Three Essays* minimize the polymorphous nature of infantile sexuality and overemphasize a maturational line leading to reproductive sexuality. Yet such fault-finding does seem unfair. After all, Freud discovered the territory and first maps of a new territory are rarely accurate.

A discussion of après-coup in sexuality generally is beyond the scope of this chapter. But we do have time to look at après-coup in connection with the origin of infantile sexuality. It's useful to return to the 20 years between 1885 and 1905. Because I am on familiar ground, I will omit a great deal.

February 1886: After four months, Freud leaves Paris seduced by Charcot's songs of hysteria and, especially, by the notion that unconscious ideas *as ideas* can cause behavior.

1886 to 1897: Whenever one dates its birth, psychoanalysis was conceived in this decade. There were major advances in technique and in theory of mind:

Technique: At first Freud used massage, diet, and suggestion to treat hysteria—the suggestion relied on his authority as a physician augmented by hypnosis. Then, influenced by Breuer's experience with Anna O., he began to look for the memory of a trauma. When he found one, he commanded the patient to forget it. Soon, hypnosis gave way to free association; the command—to forget was replaced by remembering and catharsis.

Theory of mind: Five insights formed the theoretical basis for Freud's seduction theory:

- Repression is a motivated process triggered by psychic trauma.
- Incompatible ideas are the sine qua non of psychic trauma.
- Repression is necessarily connected to sexuality.
- Two scenes, separate in time, are required for psychic trauma to lead to repression.
- The relationship between the two scenes is one of après-coup.

On September 21st, 1897, Freud wrote Fliess, "I no longer believe my neurotica." He gave four groups of reasons and then concluded:

> Now I have no idea of where I stand because I have not succeeded in gaining a theoretical understanding of repression. … It seems … arguable that only later experiences give the impetus to fantasies, which [then] hark back to childhood, and with this the factor of a hereditary disposition regains a sphere of influence from which I had made it my task to dislodge it.
>
> (1985, p. 264)

Notice that the "arguable" alternative explanation contains a combination of "hereditary disposition," which could be thought of in terms of deferred action, and "later experiences," which could be thought of in terms of retrospective modification. Many call this "abandonment of the seduction theory." As the story is usually told—including by Freud himself—Freud replaced 'seduction' with 'fantasy' and thereby founded psychoanalysis. But matters are not so simple.

What was abandoned? Only the theory that every case of hysteria was the result of a sexual seduction in childhood.

What wasn't abandoned? Everything else! The five interwoven concepts that provided the theoretical basis for the theory of seduction are

- *repression* is a motivated process triggered by psychic trauma;
- *incompatible ideas* are the sine qua non of psychic trauma;
- *repression is connected to sexuality*;
- *two scenes are required for psychic trauma to lead to repression*; and
- *the relationship between the two scenes is one of après-coup*.

It was clear to Freud that infantile sexual drives are different from non-sexual instincts; what wasn't clear was both the basis for this distinction and the origin of infantile sexuality. Freud did recognize that he had a problem. He had concluded that only a childhood experience marked as sexual can be repressed and had also concluded that childhood sexuality need not arise from seduction. He knew that if an experience is subject to repression après-coup, if it is untranslatable in the second scene, the experience must have a sexual undertone; but what is the origin of this sexual undertone and in what sense is it sexual?

What Laplanche pointed out a quarter of a century ago still holds good. Freud refused to reduce infantile sexuality to physiology and also "refused to give up the word 'sexuality' by substituting more acceptable terms like 'organ-pleasure', 'interest' and so on, [but]," writes Laplanche, "truth be told,"

among his successors even this aporia has disappeared. Because infantile, non-genital sexuality is difficult to grasp, it was quite simply abandoned. There will be reference to orality and anality, to oral and anal object relations, but hardly ever to oral or anal sexuality. These days, who among the Kleinians ever speaks of infantile sexuality? Who is concerned with pregenital erogenous pleasure? In a sense, the French ... [are] one of the last bastions of the idea of infantile sexuality.

(1990, pp. 169–170)

The question confronting Freud was, "is infantile sexuality innate or acquired?" Forced to choose one or the other, he chose both: placing innate fantasies acquired in primal times at the origin of sexuality: fantasies of seduction, castration, and parental intercourse—later on he added other fantasies. Freud might have found an alternative explanation for the origin of infantile sexuality if, instead of abandoning his seduction theory, he had generalized it as he had generalized the existence of an unconscious. Although he was not in a position to do that, he did provide two essential insights:

- repression is a failure of translation and
- après-coup is the structure of the ongoing process of repression.

Freud began to theorize après-coup in two places: the middle section of the "Project" and, a year later, in that letter to Fliess whose key phrase is "a failure of translation is known clinically as repression" (1985, p. 208). Laplanche extends this insight. He writes:

> Why then invoke a theory, a translational model of après-coup and, more generally, a translational model of the theory of seduction and even a translational model of the constitution of the human being? It is because there is no mental process that captures the double movement better than translation, the indivisible double movement of the "being carried forward" and of "referring back." The "being carried forward" is nothing other than what I designate as a "fundamental to-be-translated": a demand to translate the message of the other.
>
> (1990–1991, p. 174)

LAPLANCHE STANDING ON ONE FOOT

An attempt to summarize (some of) Laplanche's key concepts in one page

1. From birth, infants are dependent on adults in attachment relationships centered on communication; initially instinctual on the

side of the baby, on the side of the adult the communication is motivated and largely but not entirely conscious/preconscious.

2. On both sides the mental aspect—both verbal and gestural/pre-verbal—involves logical, secondary process thinking.

3. Adults have a sexual unconscious, infants do not. This asymmetry is what Laplanche calls the *fundamental anthropological situation*.

4. The adult's sexual unconscious compromises and parasitizes many of the communications with the child; in other words, it may add an enigmatic aspect to the adult's communications, enigmatic both to the adult and to the child. This enigmatic aspect is sometimes called an "enigmatic message"; *however, for the adult the enigmatic aspect* **is not** *a message* as it is not part of what is intended consciously or pre-consciously. *However, for the child the enigmatic aspect* **is** *a message* because it is recognized as addressed to the child and as having meaning for the adult.

5. The human child seeks to make sense of the adult's communications, to *translate* the communications including the enigmatic elements (!); i.e., the child is pleasantly or unpleasantly stimulated (seduced, inspired, compelled) to make sense of adult communication and the enigmatic elements which parasitize it. This is what Laplanche calls the *general theory of seduction*.

6. Precisely because the enigmatic aspects of the adult's communication are enigmatic, the child's translation can never fully succeed. The failure leaves untranslated bits, 'residues' called *designified signifiers or thing presentations*; these residues are what constitutes the repressed unconscious. This is to say, the process of (failed) translation constitutes primal repression. This is what Laplanche calls *the translational model of repression* (see Freud to Fliess Dec. 6, 1896).

7. Humans are a meaning-making species. The untranslated bits—the primally repressed—persist as a constant stimulation to repeated new attempts at translation which can never fully succeed, i.e., they are both the source and the object of meaning-making, what Laplanche calls the *source/object of the drive*.

Back to the poets. I will use Umberto Eco and Mary Gaitskill to demonstrate the richness of the connection between translation and après-coup. I'll telegraph my punch: translation is always translation of an enigmatic communication that both has an address—is seen to be addressing someone—and that has multiple potential meanings.

Near the beginning of Eco's delightful lectures, published as *Experiences in Translation* (2008), he discusses different translations of a joke in his novel *Foucault's Pendulum*. For the French and German editions, a literal translation of the Italian worked well; but translation into English was problematic, as a significant change was required to preserve the joke. Eco writes:

> Note that the English version is snappier than the Italian, and perhaps someday, on making a revised edition of my novel, I might use the English formula rather than the Italian. Would we then say that I have changed my text? We certainly would. Thus, the English translation is a failed translation of the Italian. In spite of this, the English text says exactly what I wanted to say ... a literal translation would have made the joke harder to understand.
>
> (2001, p. 8)

I mean to emphasize that translation involves seeing the text as pluripotential, as having multiple possible meanings. As I said before, each translation interacts with each previous translation to inform a new translation, a new understanding.

Now the enigmatic. What does enigmatic mean? What is the nature of the enigmatic? What is proper to the enigmatic?

Humans are a meaning-making species. The human child is confronted with adult communications and tries to make sense of them—this urge is innate. The child tries to give meaning to adult communications, to translate them, but can do so only with the cognitive and cultural tools available at a given stage of development. In most human dialog (non-verbal as well as verbal), there is no need for translation or else the translation is instantaneous; but, in adult–infant communication, when the intended meaning of the communication is compromised by the adult's sexual unconscious, the message cannot be grasped in its totality.

In other words, the entire communication addressed to the child is perceived as meaningful, including the parts marked by unconscious meanings which are, ipso facto, necessarily enigmatic. Take breast-feeding: the example psychoanalysts can't resist. Communications during breastfeeding are associated with milk and breast, with feelings of appeasement and excitation, with the 'containing' breast and the sexually exciting breast, etc. The codes the child has are insufficient for translating these associations, so the child resorts to new codes, partly improvised, partly using schemas furnished by the cultural environment. Nevertheless, some bits, some associations, remain enigmatic, untranslated—repressed. It is precisely those meanings and associations which are enigmatic, unconscious, and sexual for the adult that can never be fully or finally translated and thus are potentially a perpetual provocation to new attempts at translation.

There is a notion abroad in the land that what is enigmatic is excessive or 'too much' and, in some sense, violent. For Laplanche, the opposite is true. It is violent actions that are most likely to impose a specific meaning. Insofar as they do, they are not enigmatic, not available for translation and repression. Think of post-traumatic stress disorder (PTSD), of dreams and flashbacks that represent the trauma in unmodified form. The trauma is stuck untranslated in what Laplanche calls the enclaved unconscious. In temporal terms, it is a registration (a presentation) which precedes translation and repression, a presentation that precedes (re) presentation.

In contrast to the diamond-hard fixity of presentations in the enclaved unconscious, enigmatic representations are malleable, polysemic, open to multiple and even contradictory translations. Consider this excerpt from a story by Mary Gaitskill (1997)—a great American writer I think of as a mentor in the poetry of sadomasochism. The story's narrator recalls a woman she saw at a party the night before:

> I knew that she was divorced and that she had a young child; I thought of her at breakfast, touching her child's upturned face with her palm. I pictured the child struggling to make sense of the conflicts surging under her mother's absent, tender gesture.
>
> (1997, p. 230)

"[A] child struggling to make sense of ... conflicts surging under her mother's absent, tender gesture." It is a fine example of a child attempting to translate an enigmatic communication. The gesture is tender, not violent. It is not 'too much'; indeed, it may have a 'too little' quality as the gesture is absent as well as tender.

For a child, being caressed often involves signifiers to which no certain meaning can be assigned, enigmatic signifiers which, in the Unconscious, remain signifiers without a signification—designified signifiers. The unconscious is a collection of such designified signifiers contributed by the adult's sexual unconscious. While remaining enigmatic, they are easily associated with sexuality, they respond to sexuality in a kind of harmonic resonance.

The designified signifiers are perpetual provocations to translation; they inspire translation; they are a seduction to translation. Of course, new translations can never fully succeed because these enigmatic residues can sustain multiple and contradictory translations. Laplanche calls these residues the source-objects of the drive: "object of the drive" because they are the object of recurrent attempts at translation; "source of the drive" because they are what stimulates those recurrent attempts. Consider an inflamed splinter under your skin, or a gouty toe, or an adolescent boy's penis: touch it, even lightly, and it will demand attention. Similarly, a passing association may stimulate a de-signified signifier to demand translation. It would be more suggestive and no less precise to say that passing associations may seduce a designified signifier (or a group of them, a 'complex' of them) to demand translation.

Inverting Freud's famous formula, we could say that infantile sexual drives are a "demand for work" imposed by the mind on the body, imposed on the embodied subject by repressed, unconscious, designified signifiers activated by associations. The infantile sexual drives are drives to make meaning; they are what founds the human subject.

I conclude with a few assertions that contain each other:

- Infantile sexual drives arise from the two-step process of après-coup in which repression leaves residues of failed translations that become the source-objects of the drives and have an associative resonance with sexuality.
- These drives are a process of making meaning après-coup and are necessarily sexual because the object, the designified signifier, is marked by the caretakers' unconscious sexuality.

- Thus après-coup is at the origin of the emergence of the human subject as a sexual creature, as a self-theorizing, self-narrating creature, as a creature who desires and creates meaning.

References

Breuer, J. & Freud, S. (1893). On the psychical mechanism of hysterical phenomena. *The standard edition of the complete psychological works of Sigmund Freud, volume II* (1893–1895): Studies on hysteria, pp. 1–17.

Eco, U. (2001). *Experiences in translation* (Alastair McEwen, Trans.). Toronto: University of Toronto Press, page 8.

Freud, S. (1887–1904). *The complete letters of Sigmund Freud to Wilhelm Fliess, 1887–1904* (J. M. Masson, Trans. and Ed.). Cambridge, MA: The Belknap Press, 1985.

Freud, S. (1894). The neuro-psychoses of defense. *Standard Edition*, *3*, 47.

Freud, S. (1905). Three essays on the theory of sexuality. *Standard Edition*, 7, 219.

Gaitskill, M. (1997). *Because they wanted to: Stories* (p. 230). New York, NY: Simon & Schuster.

House, J. (2017). The ongoing rediscovery of Après-coup as a central freudian concept. *Journal of the American Psychoanalytic Association*, *65*, 773–798.

House, J. & Slotnick, J. (2015). Après-coup in French psychoanalysis: The long afterlife of nachträglichkeit. *Psychoanalytic Review*, *102*, 684–708.

Lacan, J. (1953). The function and field of speech and language in psychoanalysis. In Bruce Fink (Trans.), *Écrits* (p. 213). New York, NY: Norton, 2006.

Laplanche, J. (1987). New foundations for psychoanalysis (Jonathan House Trans.). New York, NY: The Unconscious in Translation, 2017.

Laplanche, J. (1990). Time and the other. In Luke Thurston (Trans.), *Problématiques VI: Après-coup* (pp. 169–170). New York, NY: The Unconscious in Translation, 2017.

Laplanche, J. (1990–1991). *Problématiques VI: Après-coup* (Jonathan House, Trans.). New York, NY: The Unconscious in Translation, 2017.

Laplanche, J. (2000). Drive and instinct. In John Fletcher, Jonathan House, & Nicholas Ray (Trans.). *Freud and the sexual* (p. 18). New York, NY: The Unconscious in Translation, 2011.

Laplanche, J. (2002). Starting from the fundamental anthropological situation. In John Fletcher, Jonathan House, & Nicholas Ray (Trans.). *Freud and the sexual* (pp. 99–113). New York, NY: The Unconscious in Translation, 2011.

Laplanche, J. (2003). Gender, sex, and the sexual. In John Fletcher, Jonathan House, & Nicholas Ray (Trans.), *Freud and the sexual* (p. 159). New York, NY: The Unconscious in Translation, 2011.

Laplanche, J. & Pontalis, J. B. (1964). Primal fantasy, fantasies of origin, origin of fantasy. In J. House (Trans.), *Laplanche: An introduction* (pp. 69–115.). New York, NY: The Unconscious in Translation, 2015.

Laplanche, J. & Pontalis, J. B. (1967). Deferred action; deferred. In D. Nicholson-Smith (Trans.), *The Language of psychoanalysis* (pp. 111–114). New York, NY: Norton, 1973.

Winnicott, D. (1965). Maturational processes and the facilitating environment. The International Psycho-Analytical Library, *64*, 39fn.

HOW THE WORLD BECOMES BIGGER; IMPLANTATION, INTROMISSION, AND THE APRÈS-COUP: DISCUSSION OF HOUSE

Avgi Saketopoulou

Jonathan House's conceptually rigorous paper offers us an entry point through which psychoanalysts can think through further, as psychoanalysts, about the seam between the psychic and the social. I will be focusing on some of the ideas House has clearly articulated for our benefit, with special attention to his unique contribution as to how the concept of après-coup is inextricably linked to processes of translation. House points to Laplanche's distinction between implantation and intromission; implantation, he tells us, involves "enigmatic representations [that] are malleable, polysemic, open to multiple and even contradictory translations" (p. 22). Intromission, on the other hand, involves the parent jamming specific meanings into the child, "impos[ing] a specific meaning" (p. 22), which consequently results in these "not [being] available for translation and repression" (p. 22). Using these distinctions and the work to which House puts them, I will suggest that the workings of the après-coup can help move us beyond the notion that implantations and intromissions belong to a stable conceptual grid with clearly delineated borders to suggest that these borders can become porous under some temporalizations, and, also, that both of them are conditions that earn their coherence from their historical situatedness. More specifically, House's work enables us to examine how the operation of the après-coup re-inscribes some implantations to render them traumatic. What was originally experienced as—or may have been described as—an implantation may, retroactively, be best understood, and experienced by the subject, as an intromission. To make these points, I'll build on House's example in working with textual translation, and *The Odyssey* in particular. Further, I will draw on examples from the #MeToo movement and my clinical experience to highlight some of the implications of what House's work makes possible in our thinking as analysts who live and work under particular sociopolitical conditions.

Translations: How, when, and by whom

The important question, it seems to me, is not whether a culture without restraints is possible or even desirable but whether the system of constraints in which a society functions leaves individuals the liberty to transform the system … a system of constraint becomes truly intolerable when the individuals who are affected by it don't have the means of modifying it. This can happen when such a system becomes intangible as a result of its being considered … a[n] imperative … restrictions have to be within the reach of those affected by them.

(Foucault, 1982/1983, p. 16/7)

Written nearly 3,000 years ago, Homer's *The Odyssey* has been translated into English over 60 times. Yet, only one of those is by a female scholar, Dr. Emily Wilson, a classicist at U Penn. Published in 2017, her text has been hailed as a "new cultural landmark" (Higgins, 2017), and as "scraping away all the centuries of verbal and ideological buildup" (Quinn, 2017). For reasons that will become clear shortly, I want to focus on Wilson's description of her struggle in translating one of the most notoriously difficult lines. In Homer's very first portrayal of his protagonist, Odysseus is described as an ἄνδρας πολύτροπος. The word ἄνδρας, in Greek, means 'man' while πολύτροπος is a composite word that has yielded almost as many translations as there are versions of *The Odyssey* itself,

> Chapman starts things off … with "many a way/Wound with his wisdom"; John Ogilby counters with the terser "prudent"; … [t] here's Alexander Pope's "for wisdom's various arts renown'd"; … H.F. Cary's "crafty"; … Theodore Buckley's "full of resources"; Henry Alford's "much-versed"; … George Palmer's "adventurous"; William Morris's "shifty"; … Francis Caulfeild's "restless"; Robert Hiller's "clever"; … Richmond Lattimore's "of many ways"; … Albert Cook's "of many turns"; Walter Shewring's "of wide-ranging spirit"; … Robert Fagles's "of twists and turns"; all the way to Stanley Lombardo's "cunning."
>
> (Mason, 2017)

A considerable portion of Wilson's 2017 *NY Times* interview is dedicated to what I think of as one of her most original ideas (Mason, 2017). "It is entirely defensible," she explains, "to translate the word πολύτροπος as 'straying,' and ἄνδρας not as man—as all previous male translators have done—but as 'husband' (since, in fact, ἄνδρας in Greek does also mean 'husband')." Pause for a minute to take this in: what would it mean if the recounting of Odysseus' long journey back to Ithaca were to start out with Homer appealing to the muse to help him tell the story not of a warrior, but of a straying husband? This would, no doubt, frame the remainder of this epic poem in an entirely different way[2]. When I first encountered Wilson's proposition of translating ἀνδρας πολύτροπος as "straying husband," I was stunned. I was born and raised in Greece; *The Odyssey* was part of the elementary school curriculum and I have read the text in ancient and in modern Greek a few times. Yet, while I know full well that in my native tongue ἀνδρας can mean husband just as frequently as it means man, the notion of Odysseus being first introduced to the reader as a husband—a man, that is, defined by his relationship to a woman, and a straying husband at that, had absolutely never crossed my mind. Even in reading Wilson's interview, I had to stop several times to take this in. But is this really what Homer meant, you may wonder? Wilson's translation, the *Chicago Review of Books* opines, stretches. But not beyond what is permissible (Brady, 2018). How is it, I want to ask, that it has taken more than 60 translations for such a radical translational possibility to become at all thinkable? Concretely speaking, the actual words are there in the text—this is akin to House's description of the workings of deferred action—but their particular inflection issues from Wilson's desire in the present—and this is akin to House's description of the workings of retrospective modification. Together, the two make up the après-coup. But we would be remiss if we stopped our query here, since that does not account for why it is only a woman, a feminist and an immigrant woman at that, who was able to conceive of this particular translational possibility. Put differently, what can this accumulated history of translational scotoma add to our thinking about the relationship between re-translation, après-coup, and trauma? A lot, I think, and I will now return to Laplanche's work and House's original paper to be clearer about what I am trying to say.

The crafting of translation

For Laplanche, as House eloquently explains in his paper, routine acts of parental caretaking are parasitized by the parent's sexual unconscious which inflects all communications with a surcharge for which the infant is unprepared. Implanted on the level of the psychophysiological skin, this surcharge becomes an irritant that demands attention. The infant is driven to make sense of this irritant but cannot interpret it veridically because enigmatic messages are, to begin with, unconscious to the parent him/herself (Laplanche, 1987). These messages get partly translated, helping build the ego; the untranslated remainder becomes repressed, forming the unconscious. In some instances, however, messages are not implanted but intromitted. They are, that is, delivered contentful and with an interdiction to the child to translate them in any way other than that dictated by the parent. The child, thus, cannot actively take them up to translate freely in her own improvisational way as is the case with an implantation; intromission "puts into the interior an element *resistant to all metabolization*" (Laplanche, 1999, p. 136, emphasis added). But how are translations fashioned in the first place?

The infant, Laplanche tells us, translates enigmatic messages by formatting them through the existing meaning-making templates made available to her by the parent. What are these templates? The parent conveys to the child in subtle but varied ways, most of them embodied, the surrounding culture's myths, stories, and symbols. These, in turn, become the media through which the unelaborated state of the infantile sexual can come to be invested with meaning (Laplanche, 2005). It seems to me that it is only a short step from Laplanche's assertion to argue that, since the adult (and her sexual unconscious) exist in a sociopolitical world, the translational codes she can make available to the child for translation, will by definition and necessarily be constrained by the range of myths, stories, and symbols that explicitly and implicitly order social life. Put differently, it is only the portion of the unconscious that can hook itself onto the mythosymbolic narratives widely circulating in culture, that can develop escape velocity to make it out of the inchoate so that it may be churned into some rudimentary form of meaning and, eventually, become a building block of the ego. While some creativity and improvisation are at play in the crafting of translations (Laplanche, 2006), the range of materials that we can use to translate are furnished for us by the outside, that is by our parents. In that sense, they are 'found objects' (objets trouvés; Saketopoulo, 2017), nominated for this function by the culture's existing and dominant ideologies. Laplanche comes close to this when he posits that, say, the Oedipus complex is part of the infant's self-theorizing rather than an internally derived, phylogenetically transmitted fantasy (1987). The next logical step is to conclude that nothing can exit the recesses of the unconscious if it does not hitch a ride on forms that *already exist*.

To better flesh out the implications of this sequence, I will turn to the work of Piera Aulagnier. Aulagnier (1975) proposed that the primal, raw material of the infant's early life, at the time before the I has yet even become a differentiated I, gets formatted into usable units of experience through the parent's discourse. For Aulagnier, discourse is not language per se; the term refers to the aggregate effects of how the social is structured and, in turn, structures us. Through the effects of the constant background stream of affect, acts, and words, the parent responds and names experience to and *for* the infant, and in so doing formats the amorphousness of the infant's experience, giving it a shape. Of course, all of this is inflected by the parent's own sexual unconscious, early history, and psychic conflicts; but what I am trying to emphasize here is that the parent is not an independent or sovereign agent. The parent is her/himself subject to and answerable to external regimes of organized meanings over which she/he has little control and by which she/he is saturated.

As such, the development of representations and, thus, the building of the ego is, by definition, a reproduction of the social: because of how it is constituted, representational experience stays within the contours of the discursive since it can only be midwifed into meaning by becoming formatted along the contours of what is already socially intelligible because, again, socially intelligible tools are, definitionally, the only translational possibilities that the parent can make available to the child. Aulagnier described this process as a primary violence that is exerted on the child by the parent. The word 'violence' may feel troubling and can be misleading, so let me explain what Aulagnier means. Aulagnier is not referring to physical violence; nor is she referring to explicit prohibition or an oppressive force (that is, *primary violence* is not akin to Laplanche's notion of intromission). What I understand her to mean by *violence* has to do with how the interpretative funnel that the parent provides, and through which the infant's world can take shape. That funnel is by nature restricted, and, thus, restrictive. Primary violence is best understood as placing a constraint on the most elemental level of human becoming insofar as it delimits, ahead of time, how something will become represented in the first place. It is important to emphasize that primary violence is indispensable and constitutive; its mediation is necessary if the child is going to be able to forge meaning at all.

Translations, therefore, arise from within this necessarily limited array of existing discursive frameworks that order the larger social world. That means that ways of being that have not yet entered the social and/or those which are not yet solidified in the cultural imaginary cannot become possible translational avenues. And, conversely, that a culture's most dominant meaning-making templates will more readily and widely lend themselves to becoming translational vessels. Therefore, for instance, since patriarchy, procreative heterogenitality, and binary gender are the most intelligible, socially sanctioned, and institutionally supported forms of sex and gender systems in Western culture, it should come as no surprise that they are the translational frameworks most plainly on offer.

The subject compresses all meaning into already existing shapes and if you are thinking that that's limiting, you are exactly right; there is no way around this. There is no social world without discourse or one existing outside myths or symbols. If even for a moment, and only as a thought experiment, we tried to imagine a society without such constraining structures, we would have to conclude that a social realm of this kind would actually be catastrophic. Not only would it not provide greater freedom in forging translations but, on the contrary, it would incapacitate the child since it would deprive her of any tools whatsoever with which to translate the press of the infantile sexual. The meaning-making kit of culture is all we have.

Meaning-making goes astray

Or, to immediately contradict myself, it is all we have *until we have something else*. What do I mean by that? If Wilson is able to formulate a translation of Odysseus as a straying husband, it is not because she has single-handedly been able to see what the rest of us have not. The story is a bit more complex. Her undeniable intellect and her considerable erudition are not in and of themselves sufficient. These attributes and her intellect have synergized, in this particular cultural moment, with certain discursive shifts that enable women to think with more degrees of freedom about the oppressions of patriarchy. It is this that permits Wilson, who is a feminist scholar, to escape the gravitational pull of Odysseus as a warrior to be able to deliver him to us as, also, a straying husband. It is under the auspices of such slowly accruing cultural shifts that a different set of translational forms become possible at all. New translational codes make the world bigger. The world becomes bigger every time a human society stretches to make room for more, and it becomes bigger every time it pushes against the limits of established categories. Why? On the simpler, more superficial level, because it makes room for people whose experience is not granted recognition and who have been toiling under the burdens of being unseen. But most importantly, as House's work on the après-coup of translation enables us to see, it becomes bigger because any expansion of the mytho-symbolic means that the materials through which enigma can be translated can become more varied, furnishing the subject with more possibilities for becoming. Even this expansiveness, of course, will still always be constrained since new translational tools will exert their own primary and delimiting violence, and as such, more expansion can always be possible. There is no 'final destination' for a translation; becoming also means becoming again[3], and this is, in fact, one of the most beautiful aspects of our humanity, not to mention one of the most potentially productive dimensions of the analytic work.

Such cultural shifts, however, are not just enabling of new selves; in the après-coup, they can also become traumatic because they can, retroactively, re-inscribe what had been originally registered as an implantation, rewriting it into an intromission. Here's what I mean: consider an atypically gendered subject for whom the proliferation of transgender discourses enables new translations of their gender experience, which subsequently permits them to start thinking of themselves as being transgender (as opposed to, say, an effeminate gay man or woman). This new translation can retroactively render the original implantation of the infantile sexual into gender, into an intromissive injunction: that is, where gender had initially offered a translational avenue of which the subject could avail itself (Laplanche, 2011), what was in real time an offering of translational tools may be revealed, in the après-coup, to have been subtended by binary injunctions: in other words yes, gender constituted a translational tool but only insofar as it followed the male/female binary. Some trans subjects may, thus, only retroactively come to experience the initial mandate that they arrange themselves into a neat male/female classificatory divide as traumatic. This is different than saying that the experience was traumatic all along and only became possible to register as such when a trans person came to realize that transgender life and embodiment may be viable possibilities; to say that it was traumatic all along would be a misunderstanding of après-coup as something that was already there, waiting to be discovered. What distinguishes the workings of the après-coup in this instance is that the injunction to normative gender may *become traumatic after discursive shifts of gender as multiple* have occurred. That is, it can become traumatic only after—and because of—the encounter with enlarged possibilities afforded by new translational codes around gender. Why? Because that revisitation can in the present, and considered through the lens of today's translational possibilities, restage the original implantation as an interdiction to translate gender as anything *but* binary and fixed. I am using the example of gender as an illustration to my larger point, which is this: for some subjects, cultural shifts can, in the après-coup, spin implantation into the orbit of intromission.

The scrambled temporality of the après-coup means that it is not until after cultural shifts permit the emergence of novel translational possibilities that the restrictiveness that had been affected by primary violence may come to be experienced as violent in the first place—therefore becoming traumatic after the fact. Said differently, cultural changes create translational funnels with wider translational possibilities (e.g., multiple genders rather than two, etc.) that could not have been furnished or imagined by the parent, because of the parent's cultural and historical situatedness. These new funnels can then, in turn, be taken up by the subject to translate anew, resulting in entirely different psychic positions which may render the original ones traumatic.

When culture surrenders a tight hold over reality to open up to new alternatives, primary violence, the necessary constriction that give the subject to the world, and which permits the I to move out of the primal and to start becoming, can come to be experienced in its full constrictive effects. Implantation and intromission, therefore, do not only concern the intervention of the other (the adult) on the child as Laplanche has been explicit on; they are, also, refracted through the interventions of culture and of cultural change. In other words, by considering the workings of the après-coup on translation that House has offered us, we can begin to think about implantations and intromissions as earning their coherence from their particular situatedness. We can start thinking about them, that is, as being, to some degree, historically contingent. This is not to minimize all of what we already know about how the adult implants enigmas or pressures an intromission upon a child; it is merely to say that critical to their psychic density is, also, their historical contingency.

To make what I mean by historical contingency clearer, and to close my comments, let me use an example that pertains to the #MeToo movement.[4] Imagine you are a woman in the 1990s. Or, to be more precise for the purposes of this thought experiment, imagine that you are the kind of person who identifies as—or is interpellated in terms of—the gender, class, ability, and racial background such that you could be the potential beneficiary of the cultural shifts that in 2018 will make the scenarios I describe below possible. That leaves a lot of people out, but stay with me as I try to make a point that ultimately, albeit in different ways, applies to most. Your male boss flirts with you. You try to navigate the fine line between not injuring his frail ego, keeping your job or at least not risking that raise or promotion, and not ending up intruded upon or, worse, naked. Your boss touches you flirtatiously; you discretely telegraph your unease. Maybe you were clear, maybe you were not, maybe you should have been clearer, maybe he should have been less dense, maybe he was not that dense but did not really give a damn. At the end of the day, it's more or less fine—you didn't love the experience, you felt uncomfortable, but you kept your job and, besides, you have known all along that women have to deal with this stuff all the time, that men will try to get what they can, your mother told you 'how men are' since you were a little girl, who are you to think you'd be spared such advances? But, fast forward to 2018, and in *this* particular moment in time for some women and in certain parts of the world, such behavior is no longer just ok. (Some) men are getting called out, held accountable, and your boss' actions would, perhaps, nowadays get him fired. What's different? What's different is that in the 1990s that behavior was 'men being men' while today that behavior is understood as abusive and violent. What's different is that the world has changed. Does it matter? Isn't your experience the same anyway? No, it's not. In fact, as one article after another shows up in your Facebook newsfeed informing you of this or another male executive brought down by such invasive gestures, you are finding yourself feeling more and more upset (this is the excitation of the second inscription that Freud described occurs in the second scene of the après-coup that activates the memory of the first). You find that your boss' behavior which, at the time, felt uncomfortable and annoying, now, that is, in the après-coup, is gathering speed and is beginning to feel upsetting. Your close friend reminds you that at the time, you didn't seem that disturbed—why are you getting so worked up now? The events have, after all, not changed. You know your friend is right, and you feel embarrassed and a tinge of conflicted shame. The truth is that you knew then that you could have reported your boss and you knew it was kind of illegal, and at the end of the day, you didn't really do anything about it. But, of course, what you also knew, and what all women knew, and what men did as well, was that nothing would come of it and you knew that other women also went through it, and who are you after all to think you deserved better than them? It was, in some sense, your fate as a woman to endure these intrusions. *This* is what has changed; with this cultural shift around how we are coming to see these kinds of behaviors, a new translational possibility has emerged. Then it was 'men being men'; today it is 'male violence'; today, (again, only in some parts of the world) you as a woman perhaps no longer have to take it. This, of course, continues to be mediated by your subject positionality; race, class, educational level, etc., all affect what is deemed credible reporting. But my point is that in the après-coup, that original moment of your boss touching you has now become traumatic when it may not have been so in real time.

Psychic trauma, as House has explained in laying out Freud's thinking, requires two times. From the time of original inscription and the time of its revisitation, your experience with your boss is becoming traumatic because of the particular situatedness of that moment *then in the present moment now*. For Freud, what intervened between the first inscription and the second was puberty. The child, with instinctual sexuality newly at her disposal, is returned to the original scene to which she now has a 'sexual reaction' that she didn't have before. But it's more than just puberty that can intervene between these two events. "When we speak of a sexual reaction," Laplanche writes, "we are evoking not only the possibility of new physiological reactions but, in correlate, the existence of sexual ideas" (1970, p. 39). It is these new sexual ideas that make up the discursive shifts powered by #MeToo that can offer new translational possibilities and, in turn, rewrite your uncomfortable experience into a traumatic one. And you are now able to do that because, in being able to craft this new translation, you are also able to look back and note that the 'men will be men' norm that left you then 'free' with the choice to translate what was done to you and how you wanted to go about dealing with it, now, in retrospect, is revealed to have been an intromission all along—a message that you, as woman, had to take it from the man.

The insights House has offered us in deepening our understanding of the relationship between translation and the après-coup are momentous. Their implications are far-reaching, and by no means limited to what I have begun to explore here. We should all be looking forward to tracking how they will be taken up by other analytic scholars and to the innovative analytic theorizing they can ignite in our field.

Notes

1 Adapted from Robert Fagles's prose translation; Modern Library.
2 Notably, while Wilson says, in the same interview, that such a rendering is "a viable translation," she ultimately hesitates to select it. Her hesitation issues precisely from the fact that "it would give an entirely different perspective" and an entirely different setup for the poem.
3 The ties to Deleuze are obvious, but cannot be explored here.
4 See Saketopoulou, 2018, for a more in-depth exploration of this.

Bibliography

Aulagnier, P. (1975). *The violence of interpretation: From pictogram to statement* (A. Sheridan, Trans.). Hove: Brunner-Routledge.
Brady, A. (2018). How Emily Wilson translated the Odyssey. Retrieved January 16, 2018 from https://chireviewofbooks.com/2018/01/16/how-emily-wilson -translated-the-odyssey/.
Foucault, M. (1982/1983). Sexual choice, sexual act: An interview with Michel Foucault by James O'Higgins. Salmagundi, 58/59.
Higgins, C. (2017). The Odyssey translated by Emily Wilson: A new cultural landmark. Retrieved December 7, 2017 from https://www.theguardian.com/bo oks/2017/dec/08/the-odyssey-translated-emily-wilson-review.
House, J. (this book).
Laplanche, J. (1970). *Life and death in psychoanalysis* (J. Mehlman, Trans.). Baltimore, MD: The John Hopkins.
Laplanche, J. (1987). *New foundations for psychoanalysis* (Jonathan House, Trans.). New York,NY: Unconscious in Translation.
Laplanche, J. (1999). *Essays in otherness* (J. Fletcher. Trans.). London: Routledge.
Laplanche, J. (2006). *Freud and the sexual: Essays 2000–2006* (J. Fletcher, J. House, & N. Ray. Trans.). New York, NY: International Psychoanalytic Books.
Mason, W. (2017). The first woman to translate "Odyssey" into English. Retrieved November 2, 2017 from https://www.nytimes.com/2017/11/02/magazine/the -first-woman-to-translate-the-odyssey-into-english.html.
Quinn, A. (2017). Emily Wilson's "Odyssey" scrapes the barnacles off Homer's hull. Retrieved December 2, 2017 from https://www.npr.org/2017/12/02/5677 73373/emily-wilsons-odyssey-scrapes-the-barnacles-off-homers-hull on.
Saketopoulou, A. (2017). Structured like Culture: Laplanche on the Translation of Parental Enigma. *DIVISION/Review*, 17, 51–52.
Saketopoulou, A. (2018). Using Psychoanalysis to Understand #MeToo memories. Retrieved on November 1, 2018 from https://www.nybooks.com/daily/2018/ 10/11/psychoanalysis-and-metoo-memories/.

Index

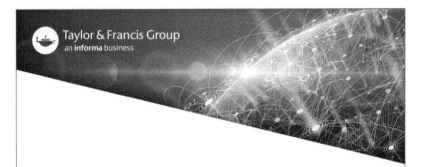

For Product Safety Concerns and Information please contact our EU
representative GPSR@taylorandfrancis.com
Taylor & Francis Verlag GmbH, Kaufingerstraße 24, 80331 München, Germany

www.ingramcontent.com/pod-product-compliance
Ingram Content Group UK Ltd.
Pitfield, Milton Keynes, MK11 3LW, UK
UKHW021439080625
459435UK00011B/312